SKIN & HAIR CARE
A Doctor's Practical Guide to Healthy Skin & Hair

Dr Prabhat Das

MD, PhD, FACP

Better Health with Dr Das Series

Hardcover ISBN: 978-1-971672-76-2

Paperback ISBN: 978-1-971672-75-5

eBook ISBN: 978-1-971672-74-8

Printed in the United States of America

Disclaimer

This book is intended solely for educational and informational purposes. It is not meant to replace personal medical advice, diagnosis, or treatment.

Although I am a licensed physician, reading this book does not establish a doctor-patient relationship. Each individual's health condition, medical history, and risk factors are unique. Any medical decision should be made in partnership with your own healthcare professional who understands your specific situation.

Medical science is continually advancing. New research and updated guidelines may lead to changes in recommendations over time.

TABLE OF CONTENTS:

About the Author 1

INTRODUCTION: Why This Book Matters.......... 4

CHAPTER 1: Why Skin and Hair Health Matters More Than You Think 10

CHAPTER 2: Understanding Your Skin — Structure, Function, and Aging 18

CHAPTER 3: Understanding Hair and Scalp — Growth, Shedding, and Loss............................ 28

CHAPTER 4: Common Warning Signs You Should Never Ignore 37

CHAPTER 5: When Skin and Hair Reflect Internal Disease 45

CHAPTER 6: What Happens When Problems Are Ignored 55

CHAPTER 7: How Doctors Diagnose Skin and Hair Problems 64

CHAPTER 8: Lifestyle That Builds Healthy Skin and Hair... 74

CHAPTER 9: Daily Skin Care Routine — Simple, Effective, and Realistic 83

CHAPTER 10: Understanding Products and Ingredients — What Works, What Doesn't, and What to Avoid... 92

CHAPTER 11: Acne — From Teenage Breakouts to Adult Struggles 102

CHAPTER 12: Dry Skin, Eczema, and Allergic Reactions — Breaking the Itch Cycle 111

CHAPTER 13: Psoriasis, Rosacea, and Chronic Skin Conditions — Learning Long-Term Control 121

CHAPTER 14: Skin Infections — Recognizing Them Early and Treating Them Right 130

CHAPTER 15: Pigmentation, Aging, and Skin Cancer Prevention — Protecting Your Skin for the Long Term 139

CHAPTER 16: Hair Loss — Causes, Patterns, and What Truly Works 151

CHAPTER 17: Scalp Disorders and Hair Care Mistakes — Fix the Root, Not Just the Hair 161

CHAPTER 18: Skin and Hair Health in Women — Understanding Hormones, Life Stages, and Real Solutions.......... 171

CHAPTER 19: Skin and Hair Health in Men — Practical Care That Works 181

CHAPTER 20: Medical, Cosmetic, and Surgical Treatments — Choosing Wisely 190

CHAPTER 21: New Research, Future Treatments, and Industry Hype — Learning to Separate Science from Marketing 200

CHAPTER 22: Frequently Asked Questions — Clear Answers to Everyday Doubts 209

CHAPTER 23: Your Lifelong Skin and Hair Health Plan — Simple Habits, Lasting Results 216

APPENDIX 1: Daily Skin and Hair Care Checklist — Keep It Simple, Keep It Consistent.......... 224

APPENDIX 2: Ingredient Guide — What Helps, What Needs Caution.......... 226

APPENDIX 3: Red Flag Symptoms — When You Should Not Wait.......... 228

APPENDIX 4: 30-Day Skin and Hair Health Plan — A Practical Start 229

APPENDIX 5: Preparing for a Doctor Visit — Make It Effective 231

Thank You and Please Review the Book..........233

Continue your Healthcare Journey with these Books 234

About the Author

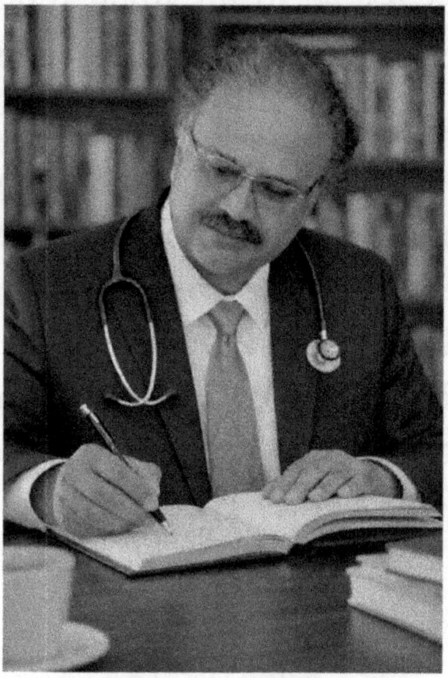

I am Dr Prabhat Das, MD, PhD, FACP. My journey in medicine began in India and, over the past thirty-five years, has continued in the United States, where I have had the privilege of caring for patients across a wide range of medical settings. I am trained in Internal Medicine, Pulmonary Diseases, and Critical Care. For me, medicine has never been just a profession. It has been a lifelong commitment shaped by learning, service, and a deep respect for the trust patients place in their physician.

Over the years, I have had the honor of caring for patients in many different situations. I have seen individuals in my office for routine concerns, treated urgent conditions in busy emergency rooms, managed serious illnesses in the hospital, and cared for critically ill patients in intensive care units. Each setting has taught me something valuable. Each patient has added to my understanding of what it truly means to care for another human being.

But one lesson has stood above all others. Medicine is not only about tests, diagnoses, or treatments. It is about people. It is about listening carefully, understanding fears that are often left unspoken, and guiding patients through uncertainty with clarity and compassion. Again and again, I have seen that what people want most is simple, trustworthy information. They want to understand what is happening in their bodies. They want to feel confident about the decisions they are making for their health and for their families.

These experiences have deeply shaped how I think about health, illness, prevention, and the human side of healing.

That is the reason behind the '**Better Health with Dr Das Series'.** Through these books, I hope to reach individuals I may never meet in person but who are searching for clear and reliable guidance. In today's world, health information is everywhere, yet much of it is confusing, overwhelming, and sometimes misleading. My goal is to cut through that noise and present important medical topics in a way that is simple, practical, and reassuring.

Every page of this series is guided by two foundations: reliable scientific knowledge and decades of real-world clinical experience. I want you, the reader, to feel informed, confident, and empowered. Not overwhelmed. Not confused. But clear about what you can do, step by step, to improve your health.

If even one reader feels less anxious, more informed, or better prepared to take control of their health after reading these books, then this work has served its purpose.

Helping people live healthier, longer, more confident and better-informed lives remains one of the greatest privileges of my life.

INTRODUCTION: Why This Book Matters

Every morning, millions of people stand before a mirror and quietly examine themselves.

A new line near the eyes.
A dark spot on the cheek.
Dryness around the mouth.
A few more hairs on the pillow.
An itchy scalp.
A rash that keeps returning.
A mole that looks slightly different.

For some people, these are small concerns. For others, they become a private worry carried through the day. Skin and hair problems can affect confidence, mood, relationships, social life, work, and the simple comfort of facing the world without self-consciousness.

This is why skin and hair health matters.

It is not merely about beauty. It is about comfort, confidence, dignity, and sometimes, important clues about health.

Skin and Hair Are Part of Whole-Body Health

The skin is the largest organ of the body. It protects us from infection, injury, sunlight, chemicals, heat, cold, and water loss. It helps regulate body temperature. It allows us to feel touch, pressure, pain, and temperature. It also works closely with the immune system.

Hair also has importance beyond appearance. It protects the scalp, reflects hormonal and nutritional changes, and carries deep personal and cultural meaning. Hair thinning or hair loss may not always be medically dangerous, but it can be emotionally painful.

As a physician, I have learned that people rarely come to the office worried only about a rash or hair loss. They often come with a deeper question: “Doctor, what is happening to me?”

That question deserves a thoughtful answer.

The Problem of Too Much Information

We live in a time when skin and hair advice is everywhere. A person can watch one video about a miracle oil, another about a collagen powder, another about a seven-step anti-aging routine, and another about a “doctor-approved” serum.

The problem is not lack of information. The problem is lack of reliable guidance.

The skin and hair care market is filled with creams, serums, shampoos, oils, supplements, devices, procedures, and promises. Some are helpful. Some are useful only for selected people. Some are exaggerated. Some may irritate the skin, delay proper diagnosis, or waste money.

A beautiful bottle does not always mean good science.
A viral video does not always mean medical truth.
A “natural” label does not always mean safe.
An expensive product does not always mean better results.

Doctor's Pearl

Good skin and hair care does not begin with buying more products. It begins with understanding the real problem.

What This Book Will Do for You

This book is written to bring clarity.

You will learn how skin works, why it becomes dry or inflamed, why acne appears, why pigmentation develops, how sun damage accumulates, and when a skin change should be checked.

You will learn how hair grows, why it sheds, what causes thinning, when hair loss may be temporary, and when early treatment is important.

You will also learn how to think about products and ingredients. What truly helps? What is overhyped? What is safe? What needs medical supervision?

Most importantly, this book will help you move away from confusion and toward confidence.

Myth vs Fact

Myth: Skin and hair problems are only cosmetic.

Fact: Some are cosmetic, but others may reflect hormones, nutrition, inflammation, infection, medications, stress, or internal disease.

Myth: Expensive products are always better.

Fact: The right product, used correctly, matters more than the price.

Myth: Natural products are always safe.

Fact: Natural substances can also irritate the skin or cause allergy.

Myth: Hair loss is always permanent.

Fact: Many types of hair loss are temporary or manageable when properly evaluated.

Common Mistakes to Avoid

Do not keep adding new products every week.

Do not believe every social media claim.

Do not ignore sudden hair loss, changing moles, painful rashes, or non-healing sores.

Do not assume every itch is allergy.

Do not use strong creams without knowing the diagnosis.

Do not expect overnight results.

Example: The Cost of Confusion

A woman in her early fifties notices dry skin and increased hair shedding. She buys an expensive shampoo, hair oil, collagen powder, and several vitamins. Months pass, but nothing improves.

When she is finally evaluated, the real issue is not shampoo. She has iron deficiency and an underactive thyroid. Once the real cause is identified, her treatment becomes clear and sensible.

This kind of story is common. It reminds us that skin and hair problems often need thoughtful evaluation, not random treatment.

Key Points

Skin and hair health affects appearance, confidence, comfort, and overall well-being.

Some skin and hair changes may reflect internal health problems.

The modern skin and hair care market contains both useful products and exaggerated claims.

Correct diagnosis is more important than random treatment.

Simple, consistent, science-based care is usually better than complicated routines.

Chapter Summary

Skin and hair are not superficial concerns. They are closely connected to health, self-image, and quality of life. The skin protects the body, responds to internal and external stress, and may show signs of disease. Hair changes may reflect aging, genetics, hormones, nutrition, illness, medications, or stress.

Modern marketing has created enormous confusion. Many people try product after product without understanding the cause of their problem. This can lead to frustration, wasted money, delayed diagnosis, and sometimes harm.

This book will guide you step by step through understanding, prevention, diagnosis, treatment, and long-term care.

Action Plan

• Look at your skin and hair concerns calmly.

• Write down your main concern.

• List all products, supplements, and treatments you currently use.

• Stop adding new products without a clear reason.

• Watch for warning signs such as changing moles, sudden hair loss, severe itching, or non-healing sores.

• Begin thinking of skin and hair care as part of whole-body health.

Bridge to Chapter 1

Before we discuss acne, hair loss, pigmentation, eczema, products, and treatments, we must first understand why skin and hair health matters so much in daily life. In the next chapter, we will begin with the big picture: why skin and hair are more than beauty, and why good information can protect both your health and your confidence.

CHAPTER 1: Why Skin and Hair Health Matters More Than You Think

The Mirror Moment

Almost every day begins the same way.

You stand in front of the mirror for a few quiet seconds. You may not even realize it, but your eyes scan your face and hair.

A little dryness around the lips.
A new dark spot.
A faint line that was not there before.
A few extra strands of hair on the sink.

You move on with your day, but that brief moment stays with you.

Over time, these small observations begin to matter more. Not because we are becoming vain, but because these changes affect how we feel about ourselves.

Skin and hair are deeply personal. They are visible to the world and quietly tied to confidence, identity, and emotional well-being.

More Than Appearance

It is easy to dismiss skin and hair concerns as cosmetic.

That is only part of the story.

Skin is a living, active organ. It protects the body from infection, injury, chemicals, sunlight, and water loss. It helps regulate temperature. It works with the immune system. It constantly repairs itself.

Hair, while often seen as cosmetic, has protective roles for the scalp and plays a powerful role in how we see ourselves.

Healthy skin feels comfortable. Healthy hair feels manageable. When something is wrong, the discomfort is not only physical. It becomes emotional.

Doctor's Pearl

If a condition changes how you feel about yourself, it deserves attention, even if it is not medically dangerous.

The Emotional Side That We Often Ignore

In clinical practice, I have seen this again and again.

A young adult with acne avoids social gatherings.
A middle-aged woman with hair thinning feels older than she is.
A man with visible skin disease becomes withdrawn.

These are not trivial concerns.

Skin and hair conditions can affect confidence, social interaction, and even professional life.

When we treat these conditions, we are not only treating the skin. We are restoring comfort and confidence.

Skin and Hair as Early Signals

One of the most important reasons to pay attention to skin and hair is this: they often reflect what is happening inside the body.

Dry skin may simply be environmental, but it may also relate to aging, thyroid problems, or other conditions.

Hair loss may be genetic, but it may also be linked to stress, illness, nutritional deficiency, or hormonal imbalance.

A dark patch on the skin may be harmless pigmentation, but in some cases, it may indicate metabolic changes.

A rash may be simple irritation, but it may also reflect infection or immune activity.

Most of these changes are not serious. But some are important signals.

Learning to recognize the difference is powerful.

Why So Many People Feel Lost

If these conditions are so common, why do so many people struggle to manage them?

The answer is simple. There is too much information, and much of it is confusing.

Every day, people are exposed to advertisements, social media advice, and product claims. One source recommends a certain routine. Another suggests the opposite. Both sound convincing.

Without clear understanding, people try one product after another. They spend money. They become frustrated.

The problem is not lack of effort. It is lack of clarity.

Doctor's Pearl

Confusion leads to over-treatment. Over-treatment leads to irritation. Irritation leads to more confusion.

The Cost of Getting It Wrong

Using the wrong approach can make things worse.

Harsh cleansers can damage the skin barrier.
Too many active ingredients can irritate the skin.
Ignoring early signs can allow problems to progress.
Delaying proper care can lead to scarring or persistent issues.

I often see patients who have tried multiple treatments without success. In many cases, a simple, correct approach would have helped much earlier.

Example: When More Becomes Less

A 50-year-old woman develops mild pigmentation on her cheeks. She begins using multiple creams recommended by friends and online sources.

Within weeks, her skin becomes irritated. The pigmentation becomes darker due to inflammation.

When she finally seeks medical advice, the first step is to stop most products, repair the skin barrier, and begin a simple, targeted plan.

Within a few months, her skin improves.

This is a common pattern. Doing more is not always better. Doing the right thing matters.

Common Mistakes to Avoid

Using too many products at the same time
Changing routines frequently
Following unverified advice
Ignoring persistent symptoms
Expecting quick results

Myth vs Fact

Myth: Skin and hair problems are only cosmetic.
Fact: They may reflect deeper health issues.

Myth: More products give better results.
Fact: Simple, consistent care is often more effective.

Myth: Hair loss is always due to aging.
Fact: Many causes are treatable or manageable.

Myth: If a product works for someone else, it will work for me.
Fact: Treatment must be individualized.

Red Flag Warnings

Seek medical advice if you notice:

- A mole that changes in size, shape, or color
- A sore that does not heal
- Sudden or patchy hair loss
- Severe or persistent itching
- Rapidly spreading rash
- Signs of infection such as pain, swelling, or pus

These signs should never be ignored.

Key Points

Skin and hair health affects both physical and emotional well-being.

They are not just cosmetic concerns.

Changes may reflect internal health.

Confusion is common due to excessive information.

Simple, correct care is often the best approach.

Chapter Summary

Skin and hair are deeply connected to health, confidence, and daily life. They are not merely cosmetic features but active parts of the body that protect, signal, and respond.

In today's world, misinformation and over-marketing have created confusion. Many people try multiple products without understanding the cause of their problem.

Recognizing the importance of skin and hair health, avoiding common mistakes, and focusing on simple, science-based care are the first steps toward better outcomes.

Action Plan

• Observe your skin and hair calmly.

• Identify your main concern.

• Avoid adding multiple new products.

• Be cautious of marketing claims.

• Watch for warning signs.

• Seek proper guidance when needed.

• Focus on simple, consistent care.

Bridge to the Next Chapter

Now that we understand why skin and hair health matters, the next step is to understand the skin itself. In the next chapter, we will explore how the skin is structured, how it functions, and why it changes with age and environment.

CHAPTER 2: Understanding Your Skin — Structure, Function, and Aging

Why Understanding Comes Before Treatment

Before choosing any cream, serum, or treatment, it is important to understand one simple truth.

Your skin is not a surface to be "fixed." It is a living, active organ.

When you understand how it works, skin care becomes simpler, more logical, and far more effective. Without that understanding, it becomes guesswork.

This chapter will give you that foundation.

The Skin Is Alive and Constantly Working

At every moment, your skin is active.

It protects you from bacteria, viruses, chemicals, sunlight, and injury. It prevents loss of water. It helps regulate temperature. It allows you to feel touch, pressure, heat, and pain.

It also repairs itself continuously.

Even when you are resting, your skin is working.

SKIN AND HAIR STRUCTURE

A simple look at the structure of skin and hair.

1. THE SKIN: THREE MAIN LAYERS

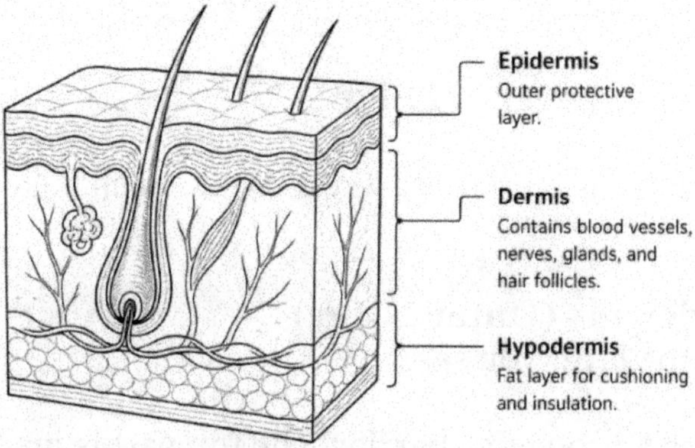

---

2. HAIR STRUCTURE

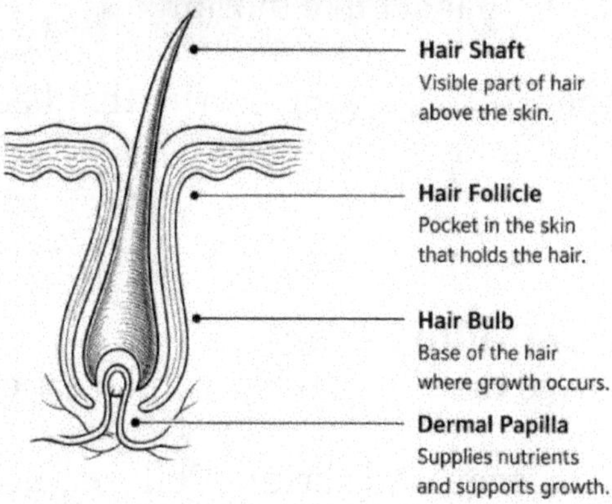

TAKEAWAY
Skin protects the body, and hair grows from follicles nourished by blood supply.

Doctor's Pearl

Healthy skin is not created by products alone. It is maintained by the skin's own natural processes.

The Three Layers of Skin

The skin is made of three main layers. Each has a specific role.

1. Epidermis (Outer Layer)
This is the layer you see.

It acts as a protective barrier. The top part is made of dead skin cells arranged like bricks. Between these cells are natural fats that act like mortar.

Together, they form a strong barrier that keeps harmful substances out and moisture in.

---

2. Dermis (Middle Layer)
This layer gives the skin strength and elasticity.

It contains collagen and elastin. Collagen provides firmness. Elastin allows the skin to stretch and return to shape.

It also contains blood vessels, nerves, hair follicles, and glands.

---

3. Subcutaneous Layer (Deep Layer)
This layer contains fat and connective tissue.

It cushions the body, provides insulation, and gives shape to the skin.

Why the Skin Barrier Matters So Much

Among all these structures, one concept is central to skin care: the skin barrier.

When the barrier is healthy, the skin feels smooth, comfortable, and balanced.

When the barrier is damaged, the skin becomes dry, sensitive, and easily irritated.

Many common problems begin here.

Harsh soaps, excessive washing, hot water, strong exfoliants, and too many active products can damage the barrier.

Environmental factors such as cold weather and aging also weaken it.

Doctor's Pearl

If your skin is irritated, the first step is not stronger treatment. It is barrier repair.

Oil, Sweat, and Balance

The skin produces oil through sebaceous glands.

This oil keeps the skin soft and flexible.

Too much oil may contribute to acne. Too little oil leads to dryness.

Sweat helps regulate body temperature.

The goal is not to remove oil or sweat completely. The goal is balance.

The Skin Microbiome

Your skin is home to many microorganisms.

This is normal.

These organisms help maintain balance and protect against harmful bacteria.

Over-cleansing or harsh treatments may disturb this balance.

Healthy skin is not sterile. It is balanced.

Why Skin Becomes Dry or Sensitive

Dry skin is very common, especially with age.

As we grow older, the skin produces less oil and holds less moisture.

Cold weather, low humidity, and frequent washing worsen dryness.

Sensitive skin often reflects a weak barrier.

When the barrier is damaged, the skin reacts more easily to products, temperature changes, and environmental exposure.

Inflammation: A Common Pathway

Many skin problems share a common feature: inflammation.

Inflammation may appear as redness, swelling, itching, or irritation.

In lighter skin, it often looks red. In darker skin, it may appear darker, purplish, or thickened.

Recognizing inflammation is important, even when it looks different.

How Aging Changes the Skin

Aging affects every layer of the skin.

The outer layer becomes thinner and repairs more slowly.

The middle layer loses collagen and elastin, leading to wrinkles and reduced firmness.

Oil production decreases, causing dryness.

Healing becomes slower.

Sun exposure accelerates these changes. This is known as photoaging.

Doctor's Pearl

Daily sun protection is one of the most effective ways to slow visible aging.

Common Mistakes to Avoid

Using very hot water
Over-exfoliating
Using multiple strong products
Ignoring dryness and irritation
Trying to correct every minor change

These habits often worsen skin problems.

Myth vs Fact

Myth: Dry skin means you are not drinking enough water.
Fact: Most dryness is due to barrier problems.

Myth: Oily skin does not need moisturizer.
Fact: All skin types need proper hydration.

Myth: Tingling means a product is working.
Fact: It often means irritation.

Myth: Scrubbing improves skin health.
Fact: It damages the barrier.

Red Flag Warnings

Seek medical advice if you notice:

- A sore that does not heal
- Persistent irritation
- Painful or blistering skin
- Rapidly spreading rash
- Unusual skin changes

Example: Too Much Treatment

A 48-year-old woman begins using multiple products for aging and pigmentation.

Within weeks, her skin becomes red, dry, and sensitive.

The issue is not lack of treatment. It is over-treatment.

When she simplifies her routine and focuses on barrier repair, her skin improves.

Key Points

The skin is a complex, active organ.

It has three layers with specific roles.

The skin barrier is essential for protection.

Oil, sweat, and microbiome maintain balance.

Aging and environment affect skin health.

Chapter Summary

Understanding the structure and function of the skin is the foundation of effective care. The skin is not just a surface. It is a living organ with protective, sensory, and regulatory roles.

The skin barrier is central to maintaining comfort and health. Many problems arise when this barrier is damaged.

Aging, environment, and improper care can affect the skin, but simple, consistent habits can support its function.

Action Plan

- Use gentle cleansing methods.
- Avoid hot water and harsh scrubbing.
- Moisturize regularly.
- Protect your skin from sun exposure.
- Keep your routine simple.
- Observe how your skin responds.
- Focus on balance, not extremes.

Bridge to the Next Chapter

Now that we understand the skin, the next step is to understand hair and scalp. In the next chapter, we will explore how hair grows, why it sheds, and what changes should not be ignored.

CHAPTER 3: Understanding Hair and Scalp — Growth, Shedding, and Loss

When Hair Begins to Change

Hair changes rarely happen overnight.

At first, it is subtle. A few extra strands on the pillow. A little more hair in the shower. A wider part that you did not notice before. A slightly thinner ponytail.

You may ignore it for weeks or months. Then one day, it becomes difficult to ignore.

Hair is closely tied to identity. It reflects age, genetics, hormones, and overall health. That is why even small changes can feel significant.

To manage hair problems well, we must first understand how hair grows and why it sheds.

Hair Is Alive at the Root, Not at the Tip

Each hair grows from a tiny structure called a hair follicle, located within the skin.

The visible part of hair, the shaft, is made of keratin. It is not alive. That is why cutting hair does not hurt.

The living part is deep in the follicle. At the base is the hair bulb, where cells divide and grow. These cells push the hair upward.

Each follicle also has an oil gland that produces natural oil, helping keep hair soft and flexible.

Doctor's Pearl

Hair care products affect the hair shaft. Hair growth is controlled at the follicle.

The Hair Growth Cycle

Hair does not grow continuously. It follows a cycle.

Growth Phase (Anagen)
This phase lasts several years. Hair actively grows during this time.

Transition Phase (Catagen)
This is a short phase when growth slows.

Resting and Shedding Phase (Telogen)
Hair rests and eventually sheds. A new hair begins to grow from the same follicle.

At any time, most hairs are growing, while a smaller number are shedding.

HAIR GROWTH CYCLE

Hair grows in a cycle of four natural stages.

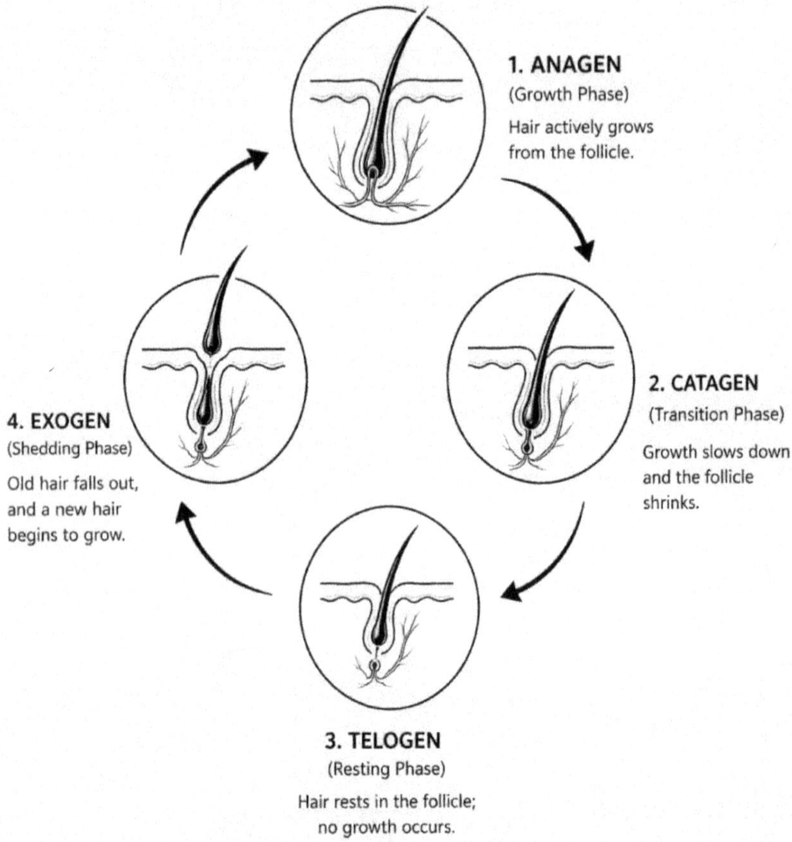

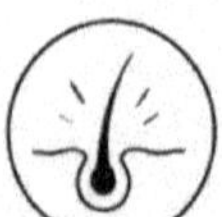

TAKEAWAY

Healthy hair grows, rests, and sheds in a continuous cycle. This cycle keeps your hair naturally renewing.

What Is Normal Hair Loss

It is normal to lose about 50 to 100 hairs per day.

These hairs are replaced by new growth.

Seeing hair on your comb or in the shower does not automatically mean something is wrong.

Concern arises when:

Shedding increases noticeably
Hair becomes thinner
The scalp becomes more visible
Hair falls out in patches

Doctor's Pearl

Do not panic over daily hair shedding. Pay attention to patterns and change over time.

Common Causes of Hair Loss

Hair loss has many causes. Understanding the pattern helps identify them.

Pattern Hair Loss
This is the most common type. It develops gradually and is influenced by genetics and hormones. In men, it leads to a receding hairline and thinning at the crown. In women, it causes overall thinning on the top of the scalp.

Telogen Effluvium
This causes sudden increase in hair shedding. It usually occurs a few months after stress, illness, surgery, childbirth, or rapid weight loss.

Alopecia Areata
This causes patchy hair loss. It is related to the immune system.

Nutritional and Hormonal Causes
Iron deficiency, thyroid disorders, and hormonal imbalance can affect hair growth.

The Scalp: The Soil for Hair Growth

Healthy hair requires a healthy scalp.

The scalp is skin. It can develop dryness, inflammation, infection, or scaling.

Dandruff, psoriasis, fungal infections, and irritation can all affect the scalp.

When the scalp is inflamed or unhealthy, hair growth may be affected.

Daily Hair Care: Small Habits Matter

Many hair problems are influenced by daily habits.

Excessive heat from dryers or straighteners weakens hair.

Tight hairstyles pull on follicles and may lead to hair loss over time.

Frequent chemical treatments damage the hair shaft.

Gentle handling, mild products, and proper conditioning help maintain hair strength.

Hair Oils: What They Can and Cannot Do

Hair oils are widely used.

They can improve dryness and shine.

They can reduce friction and breakage.

However, they do not treat most causes of hair loss.

Understanding this prevents unrealistic expectations.

Common Mistakes to Avoid

Panic over normal shedding
Switching products frequently
Using excessive heat or chemicals
Tight hairstyles
Expecting quick results

Myth vs Fact

Myth: Washing hair causes hair loss.
Fact: It removes hair that is already shedding.

Myth: Cutting hair makes it grow faster.
Fact: Growth occurs at the root.

Myth: Oils can cure hair loss.
Fact: They improve hair texture, not all causes.

Myth: Hair loss is always permanent.
Fact: Many types are temporary or manageable.

Red Flag Warnings

Seek medical advice if you notice:

- Sudden heavy shedding
- Patchy hair loss
- Hair loss with scalp pain or redness
- Hair loss with fatigue or weight change
- Loss of eyebrows or body hair

Example: Stress and Hair Loss

A 45-year-old man recovers from a serious illness. Two months later, he notices increased hair shedding.

This delayed shedding is typical of stress-related hair loss.

With time, as the body recovers, hair growth returns.

Understanding this pattern reduces anxiety.

Key Points

Hair grows in cycles.

Daily shedding is normal.

Patterns help identify causes.

Scalp health is essential.

Gentle care supports stronger hair.

Chapter Summary

Hair growth follows a natural cycle of growth, transition, and shedding. Some daily hair loss is normal, but increased shedding or thinning may indicate a problem.

Hair loss may result from genetics, stress, illness, nutritional deficiency, hormonal changes, or scalp conditions.

Understanding the pattern of hair loss and maintaining scalp health are essential for proper care.

Action Plan

- Observe your hair pattern calmly.
- Note recent stress, illness, or weight change.
- Avoid tight hairstyles and excessive heat.
- Use gentle hair care.
- Do not overload hair with products.
- Seek medical advice for unusual hair loss.
- Be patient. Hair growth takes time.

Bridge to the Next Chapter

Now that we understand how hair grows and sheds, the next step is to recognize early warning signs. In the next chapter, we will focus on common symptoms, what they mean, and when they should not be ignored.

CHAPTER 4: Common Warning Signs You Should Never Ignore

Learning to Notice What Matters

The body rarely becomes unwell without giving signals.

Skin and hair are often the first places where these signals appear. A small rash, a persistent itch, a patch of hair loss, a mole that slowly changes. These signs are easy to overlook, especially when they are mild in the beginning.

The purpose of this chapter is not to create worry. It is to help you become observant in a calm and sensible way.

When you recognize patterns early, you avoid unnecessary delay and prevent complications.

Itching: A Symptom, Not a Diagnosis

Almost everyone experiences itching at some time.

Occasional itching from dryness, weather, or minor irritation is common.

However, persistent itching deserves attention.

It may be caused by dry skin, eczema, allergic reactions, infections, or inflammatory conditions. In some cases, especially when there is no visible rash, it may be related to internal conditions.

Night-time itching, widespread itching, or itching that does not improve with simple care should be evaluated.

Doctor's Pearl

If itching continues despite simple care, look for the cause rather than trying more products.

Rashes: Patterns Tell the Story

A rash is not a single disease. It is a description.

Rashes can appear as redness, bumps, scaling, patches, or blisters.

The pattern provides important clues.

Location matters. A rash in skin folds suggests a different cause than a rash on exposed areas.

Shape matters. A ring-shaped rash may suggest fungal infection.

Duration matters. A rash that appears suddenly may differ from one that persists for months.

A rash that spreads quickly, becomes painful, or is associated with fever should not be ignored.

Acne That Persists or Worsens

Acne is common, but not all acne behaves the same.

New acne in adulthood, especially along the jawline, often has a hormonal pattern.

Acne that becomes painful, widespread, or leaves marks needs attention.

Early treatment helps prevent scarring.

Pigmentation and Color Changes

Changes in skin color are common and often harmless.

Dark spots may follow acne, injury, or irritation.

However, sudden or unusual pigmentation changes should be observed carefully.

Darkening in certain areas, such as the neck or skin folds, may reflect metabolic changes.

Uneven facial pigmentation may be related to sun exposure or hormonal factors.

Most pigmentation is not dangerous, but patterns matter.

Hair Loss: When It Needs Attention

Hair shedding is normal, but certain patterns require evaluation.

Sudden increase in hair fall
Gradual thinning over time
Patchy hair loss
Loss of eyebrows or body hair

These changes may reflect stress, illness, hormonal imbalance, or other conditions.

Nail Changes: Small but Important Clues

Nails often reflect internal and skin health.

Changes such as pitting, discoloration, thickening, or brittleness may be linked to skin diseases, infections, or nutritional issues.

Persistent nail changes should not be ignored.

Non-Healing Sores and Growths

One of the most important warning signs is a lesion that does not heal.

Any sore that persists, bleeds, crusts, or gradually enlarges needs evaluation.

These changes may be minor, but they may also represent serious conditions if ignored.

Doctor's Pearl

A skin change that persists is always more important than one that appears briefly and disappears.

Pattern and Duration: Two Key Clues

In medicine, pattern and duration guide diagnosis.

A symptom that appears briefly and resolves is usually less concerning.

A symptom that persists, spreads, or changes over time needs attention.

Observing these details makes a significant difference.

Common Mistakes to Avoid

Ignoring persistent symptoms
Assuming every rash is allergy
Delaying evaluation
Using multiple treatments without diagnosis
Expecting quick improvement

These habits delay proper care.

Myth vs Fact

Myth: If a rash is not painful, it is harmless.
Fact: Many serious conditions are painless initially.

Myth: Hair loss is always due to age.
Fact: Many causes are treatable.

Myth: Dark spots are always harmless.
Fact: Most are, but some need evaluation.

Myth: Itching is always due to dryness.
Fact: It has many possible causes.

Red Flag Warnings

Seek medical advice if you notice:

- A mole that changes in size, shape, or color
- A sore that does not heal
- Sudden or patchy hair loss
- Severe or persistent itching
- Rapidly spreading rash
- Rash with fever
- Painful or blistering skin lesions
- Unexplained skin thickening

Example: A Missed Signal

A 60-year-old man notices a small lesion on his cheek that does not heal. He assumes it is minor irritation.

Over several months, the lesion enlarges and begins to bleed.

Evaluation later reveals a skin cancer that could have been treated earlier.

This example shows the importance of early attention.

Key Points

Skin and hair often give early warning signs.

Persistent symptoms need evaluation.

Pattern and duration are important clues.

Early attention prevents complications.

Chapter Summary

Skin and hair changes often provide early signals of underlying problems. Itching, rashes, acne, pigmentation changes, hair loss, nail changes, and non-healing sores are common warning signs.

Most of these are harmless, but some require attention.

Recognizing patterns, duration, and associated symptoms helps in deciding when to seek care.

Action Plan

- Observe changes without panic.
- Note when symptoms started.
- Watch for patterns and triggers.
- Avoid self-diagnosing complex problems.
- Seek medical advice for persistent symptoms.
- Act early when warning signs appear.
- Stay calm and informed.

Bridge to the Next Chapter

Now that you can recognize warning signs, the next step is to understand what they may represent inside the body. In the next chapter, we will explore how skin and hair can reflect internal health conditions.

CHAPTER 5: When Skin and Hair Reflect Internal Disease

Looking Beyond the Surface

Most skin and hair problems are local. A new soap causes irritation. Weather leads to dryness. Blocked pores lead to acne.

But sometimes, the story is deeper.

The skin and hair can act as early messengers. They may reveal changes happening inside the body before other symptoms become obvious.

The goal is not to become anxious. It is to become thoughtful.

When you see skin and hair in the context of whole-body health, your decisions become clearer and more effective.

The Skin as a Window to the Body

The skin is closely connected to many internal systems.

It responds to changes in hormones, metabolism, nutrition, immunity, and circulation.

When something is out of balance, the skin may show:

Dryness
Color changes

Rashes
Itching
Delayed healing

Hair behaves in a similar way. It responds to stress, illness, nutritional status, and hormonal changes.

Most changes are not serious. But patterns and associated symptoms matter.

Doctor's Pearl

When skin or hair changes occur along with fatigue, weight change, or other symptoms, always think of the whole body.

Thyroid Disorders

The thyroid gland plays a major role in metabolism.

In an underactive thyroid, the skin may become dry, rough, and cold. Hair may become coarse, brittle, and thin. There may be loss of the outer part of the eyebrows.

In an overactive thyroid, the skin may feel warm and moist. Hair may become fine and may shed more easily.

These changes are often accompanied by fatigue, weight change, or changes in heart rate.

WHEN SKIN AND HAIR REFLECT INTERNAL DISEASE

Your skin and hair can show what's happening inside your body.

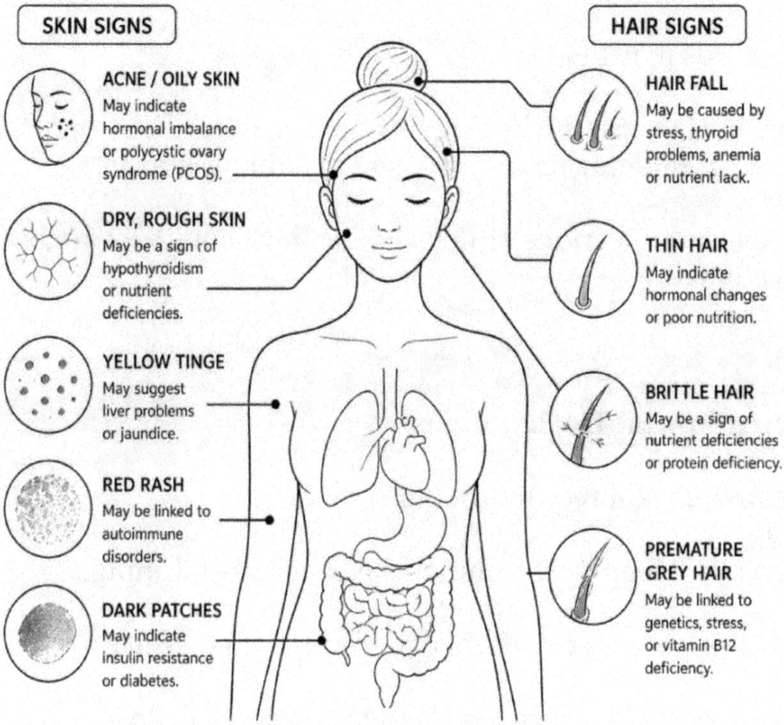

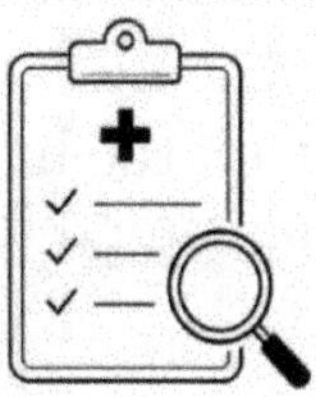

TAKEAWAY

Changes in your skin and hair can be early clues of internal health issues.

Listen to the signs. Check the cause. Take care early.

Diabetes and Skin Clues

Diabetes can affect the skin in multiple ways.

Dry skin is common. There may be frequent infections, especially fungal infections in skin folds.

Wounds may heal slowly.

Darkening and thickening of skin in areas such as the neck or underarms may suggest insulin resistance.

Repeated infections or delayed healing should always be evaluated.

Nutritional Deficiencies

Hair and skin require proper nutrition.

Iron deficiency is a common cause of hair thinning.

Protein deficiency affects hair strength and growth.

Vitamin deficiencies may lead to brittle hair, slow healing, or skin changes.

Rapid weight loss or strict dieting can disrupt the hair growth cycle, leading to increased shedding after a few months.

Balanced nutrition is essential.

Hormonal Imbalance

Hormones influence oil production, pigmentation, and hair growth.

Hormonal acne often appears along the jawline.

Certain conditions may cause acne, increased facial hair, and scalp hair thinning.

Pigmentation changes such as melasma may also be influenced by hormones.

Menopause can lead to dry skin and thinning hair.

Stress and Illness

Stress has real physical effects.

After illness, surgery, or emotional stress, many hair follicles may enter the shedding phase.

This leads to noticeable hair loss after a delay of a few months.

This type of hair loss is usually temporary, but it can be distressing.

Understanding this pattern helps reduce anxiety.

Autoimmune Conditions

In some conditions, the immune system affects the body's own tissues.

This may lead to:

Psoriasis, with thick scaly patches
Alopecia areata, with patchy hair loss
Other rashes or sensitivity to sunlight

These conditions often require medical evaluation and ongoing care.

Liver, Kidney, and Systemic Conditions

Certain internal diseases can show clear signs on the skin.

Yellowing of the skin or eyes may indicate liver problems.

Severe itching without rash may be related to liver or kidney disease.

Unusual bruising or swelling may also reflect systemic illness.

These signs are less common but important.

Common Mistakes to Avoid

Ignoring associated symptoms
Treating only the surface problem

Using supplements without clear need
Delaying evaluation

These habits can delay diagnosis.

Myth vs Fact

Myth: Skin problems are always local.
Fact: Some reflect internal disease.

Myth: Hair loss is only cosmetic.
Fact: It may signal health issues.

Myth: Supplements fix most hair problems.
Fact: They help only when deficiency exists.

Myth: Stress affects only the mind.
Fact: It affects the body as well.

Red Flag Warnings

Seek medical advice if you notice:

- Hair loss with fatigue or weight change
- Recurrent infections
- Yellowing of skin or eyes
- Severe itching without rash
- Sudden widespread skin changes
- Darkening of skin folds
- Slow-healing wounds

Example: A Hidden Cause

A 55-year-old woman develops dry skin and hair thinning. She assumes it is aging.

She also feels tired but ignores it.

Evaluation reveals an underactive thyroid.

With treatment, her energy improves, and hair shedding decreases.

This example shows how skin and hair can reflect internal health.

Key Points

Skin and hair are connected to overall health.

Hormones, nutrition, and stress influence them.

Some diseases show early signs on the skin.

Patterns and associated symptoms are important.

Chapter Summary

Skin and hair changes are not always isolated problems. They may reflect deeper processes such as hormonal imbalance, nutritional deficiency, metabolic disease, autoimmune conditions, or stress.

Understanding these connections helps avoid treating only the surface.

Recognizing patterns and associated symptoms leads to timely diagnosis and better outcomes.

Action Plan

• Observe changes in context of your overall health.

• Note associated symptoms such as fatigue or weight change.

• Maintain balanced nutrition.

• Avoid unnecessary supplements.

• Seek medical advice when multiple symptoms are present.

• Do not ignore persistent or unusual changes.

• Think of skin and hair as part of whole-body health.

Bridge to the Next Chapter

Now that we understand how skin and hair can reflect internal disease, the next step is to understand what happens when these problems are ignored. In the next chapter, we will explore complications and why timely care is so important.

CHAPTER 6: What Happens When Problems Are Ignored

Small Problems Rarely Stay Small

Most skin and hair concerns do not begin dramatically.

They start quietly.

A little dryness.
Mild acne.
Occasional itching.
Slight thinning of hair.

Because these changes seem minor, many people ignore them. Some try random products. Others wait, hoping the problem will settle on its own.

Sometimes it does. But often, it does not.

What could have been managed early and simply may slowly become more persistent, more visible, and sometimes more difficult to treat.

This chapter is not meant to alarm you. It is meant to help you understand why timely attention matters.

The Skin Barrier Breakdown

One of the earliest consequences of neglect or incorrect treatment is damage to the skin barrier.

When the barrier is weakened, the skin loses moisture and becomes more sensitive.

You may notice:

Dryness
Tightness
Burning or stinging
Increased reaction to products

Many people respond by adding more treatments.
Stronger cleansers, multiple creams, frequent exfoliation.

This often worsens the problem.

The skin enters a cycle of irritation and sensitivity.

Doctor's Pearl

When the skin becomes sensitive, reduce, do not increase, your treatment.

From Irritation to Chronic Inflammation

Repeated irritation can lead to ongoing inflammation.

Over time, this may result in chronic conditions such as dermatitis or eczema.

The skin may become:

Red or darker
Thickened
Itchy
Sensitive

Flare-ups become more frequent.

Early care can often prevent this progression.

Infection: When the Barrier Is Broken

Damaged skin is more vulnerable to infection.

Scratching itchy skin creates small openings.

Bacteria or fungi can enter and multiply.

Acne that is repeatedly squeezed may become infected.

Fungal infections may spread if not treated properly.

In people with conditions such as diabetes, even minor infections can become more significant.

Recognizing early signs such as redness, warmth, swelling, or discharge is important.

Scarring and Long-Term Changes

Some conditions leave lasting marks if not treated early.

Acne may lead to permanent scars.

Repeated inflammation may cause dark spots or uneven pigmentation.

Chronic scratching may thicken and darken the skin.

These changes are often much harder to treat than the original problem.

Prevention is always easier than correction.

Hair Loss: When Delay Matters

Hair loss often begins gradually.

In some cases, early treatment can slow or limit progression.

If ignored, certain types may advance and become more noticeable.

Some inflammatory scalp conditions may damage hair follicles if untreated.

Tight hairstyles over long periods may lead to traction hair loss that becomes permanent.

Recognizing early patterns makes a difference.

The Emotional Impact Builds Over Time

Skin and hair problems do not remain purely physical.

Visible changes may affect confidence and social comfort.

Persistent problems may lead to frustration or withdrawal.

Many people feel they should ignore these concerns. But over time, they become more distressing.

Addressing problems early helps both physical and emotional well-being.

Delayed Diagnosis of Important Conditions

Some serious conditions begin with subtle signs.

A changing mole
A non-healing sore
Repeated infections
Persistent itching without rash

If these are ignored, diagnosis is delayed.

Early treatment becomes more difficult.

Doctor's Pearl

A problem that does not improve deserves attention, even if it seems minor.

The Cost of Trial and Error

Many people try multiple products without understanding the cause of their condition.

They change routines frequently.

They follow advice from advertisements or social media.

This trial-and-error approach often leads to:

Wasted time
Unnecessary expense
Worsening symptoms

A clear diagnosis and a simple plan are usually more effective.

Common Mistakes to Avoid

Ignoring persistent symptoms
Overusing products
Picking or scratching lesions
Delaying medical evaluation
Relying only on online advice

Myth vs Fact

Myth: Skin problems will resolve on their own.
Fact: Many need proper care.

Myth: More treatment gives faster results.
Fact: Over-treatment causes damage.

Myth: Hair loss is always temporary.
Fact: Some types progress over time.

Myth: If it is not painful, it is not serious.
Fact: Many conditions are painless initially.

Red Flag Warnings

Seek medical advice if you notice:

- A sore that does not heal
- Rapidly worsening rash
- Signs of infection
- Persistent or worsening hair loss
- Changing moles or growths
- Severe itching

Example: Preventable Scarring

A young adult develops acne but does not seek treatment. He frequently picks at the lesions.

Over time, the acne settles, but scars remain.

These scars become a long-term concern and are more difficult to treat.

Early care could have prevented this outcome.

Key Points

Small problems can become more significant if ignored.

Barrier damage leads to ongoing irritation.

Infections may develop in damaged skin.

Scarring and pigmentation changes may be long-lasting.

Hair loss may progress over time.

Chapter Summary

Skin and hair problems often begin as minor concerns. When ignored or treated incorrectly, they may progress into more persistent or complex conditions.

Barrier damage, infection, scarring, pigmentation changes, and progressive hair loss are common consequences.

Early attention, correct diagnosis, and simple, consistent care can prevent many of these outcomes.

Action Plan

- Do not ignore persistent symptoms.
- Avoid using multiple treatments at once.
- Protect your skin barrier.
- Avoid picking or scratching.
- Watch for warning signs.
- Seek medical advice when needed.
- Act early rather than late.

Bridge to the Next Chapter

Now that we understand why early attention matters, the next step is to understand how doctors identify these problems accurately. In the next chapter, we will explore how skin and hair conditions are diagnosed and why correct diagnosis makes all the difference.

CHAPTER 7: How Doctors Diagnose Skin and Hair Problems

Clarity Before Treatment

One of the most common reasons people do not improve is simple.

The diagnosis is not clear.

A rash is labeled as "allergy" without proper evaluation. Hair loss is dismissed as "age." Acne is treated with random products. When the cause is uncertain, even good treatments fail.

In medicine, everything begins with diagnosis.

When the cause is understood, treatment becomes simpler, more precise, and more effective.

It Begins with a Conversation

Good diagnosis often starts with listening.

A doctor will ask when the problem began, how it has changed, and what makes it better or worse.

Important questions include:

When did this start
Did it appear suddenly or gradually
Is it improving, worsening, or unchanged
Any recent illness, stress, or weight change
Any new products, soaps, or medications
Any similar problem in the past
Family history

For hair problems, timing is especially important. Hair shedding that begins a few months after stress or illness often follows a typical pattern.

For skin problems, exposure to new products, environmental factors, or occupation may provide important clues.

Doctor's Pearl

The history often gives half the diagnosis. The skin and scalp provide the rest.

The Power of Observation

Dermatology relies heavily on careful observation.

The doctor examines:

Location
Shape
Color
Texture
Distribution

These details provide valuable information.

For example:

A rash in skin folds suggests a different cause than one on exposed areas.

A ring-shaped lesion may suggest fungal infection.

Scaling on the scalp may indicate dandruff, psoriasis, or fungal disease.

Hair examination includes:

Density
Thickness
Pattern of loss
Scalp condition

Nails are also examined, as they may provide additional clues.

Simple Office Tests

In many cases, simple tests help confirm the diagnosis.

A hair pull test may be done to assess active shedding.

A skin scraping may be examined for fungal infection.

Magnification tools may be used to examine the skin more closely.

These tests are quick and usually painless.

Blood Tests: When Needed

Not every condition requires blood tests.

However, when internal causes are suspected, certain tests may be useful.

These may include:

Thyroid function tests
Iron levels
Blood sugar
Blood counts
Hormonal tests in selected cases

Tests are chosen based on suspicion, not done routinely.

Skin Biopsy: Looking Deeper

When the diagnosis is uncertain, a biopsy may be recommended.

A small sample of skin is taken under local anesthesia.

It is then examined under a microscope.

This helps confirm diagnosis and differentiate similar conditions.

Biopsy is especially useful in unclear rashes or suspected serious conditions.

Patch Testing for Allergies

When repeated rashes occur, especially in areas exposed to products, contact allergy may be suspected.

Patch testing helps identify specific triggers.

Small amounts of substances are applied to the skin and observed over time.

Identifying and avoiding the trigger often leads to improvement.

When to See a Specialist

Many mild conditions can be managed with basic care.

However, certain situations require specialist evaluation:

Persistent symptoms
Unclear diagnosis
Severe conditions
Lack of response to treatment

Specialists have additional tools and experience for complex cases.

HOW DIAGNOSIS IS MADE FOR HAIR AND SKIN

A step-by-step approach helps find the true cause.

1. MEDICAL HISTORY

Your doctor asks about symptoms, duration, medical conditions, medications, diet, stress and family history.

2. PHYSICAL EXAMINATION

Doctor examines your skin and scalp, and looks for signs such as rash, scaling, hair loss pattern, or lesions.

3. LABORATORY TESTS

Blood or other tests may be done to check for hormonal imbalance, nutrient deficiencies, infection or allergies.

4. SPECIAL TESTS

Scalp biopsy, skin scraping, fungal culture, or trichoscopy may be done for a detailed assessment.

5. DIAGNOSIS & PLAN

Your doctor identifies the cause and creates a personalized treatment plan for you.

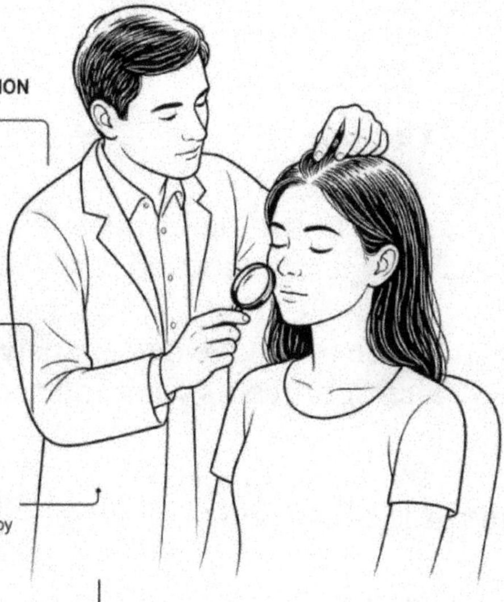

TAKEAWAY

Accurate diagnosis is the first step to effective treatment and healthy skin and hair.

Right diagnosis. Right treatment. Better results.

Common Mistakes to Avoid

Self-diagnosing based on images
Using strong treatments without diagnosis
Delaying consultation
Expecting instant answers
Not sharing complete information

These mistakes delay proper care.

Myth vs Fact

Myth: All skin problems need lab tests.
Fact: Many are diagnosed clinically.

Myth: More tests give better answers.
Fact: The right test is what matters.

Myth: Biopsy is dangerous.
Fact: It is a safe and useful tool.

Myth: Hair loss always needs extensive testing.
Fact: Many cases are diagnosed by history and examination.

Red Flag Warnings

Seek medical advice if you notice:

- Rapidly changing skin lesions
- Non-healing sores

- Severe or spreading rash
- Painful or blistering skin
- Sudden patchy hair loss
- Recurrent infections

Example: The Wrong Assumption

A man develops an itchy rash and assumes it is allergy. He uses multiple creams without improvement.

On evaluation, the pattern suggests fungal infection. A simple test confirms it.

With correct treatment, the rash improves quickly.

This example shows how similar-looking problems may have different causes.

Key Points

Diagnosis is the foundation of treatment.

History and examination provide most answers.

Simple tests confirm the diagnosis.

Blood tests are used selectively.

Accurate diagnosis prevents unnecessary treatment.

Chapter Summary

Diagnosing skin and hair problems requires careful history and examination. Additional tests are used when needed to confirm the diagnosis.

Understanding this process helps avoid confusion and unnecessary treatments.

Correct diagnosis leads to better outcomes and simpler care.

Action Plan

- Do not start multiple treatments without understanding the cause.
- Observe timing and triggers.
- Keep a simple record of symptoms.
- Seek medical advice for persistent problems.
- Share complete and accurate information.
- Follow recommended tests when needed.
- Focus on correct diagnosis.

Bridge to the Next Chapter

Now that we understand how diagnosis is made, the next step is to understand how daily lifestyle influences skin and hair health. In the next chapter, we will explore the role of diet, sleep, stress, and daily habits.

CHAPTER 8: Lifestyle That Builds Healthy Skin and Hair

The Quiet Power of Daily Habits

When people think about improving their skin or hair, they often look for a new product.

A better cream. A stronger serum. A special shampoo.

But in my experience, the most meaningful improvements do not begin in a bottle. They begin with daily habits.

What you eat, how you sleep, how you manage stress, and how you live each day quietly shape your skin and hair over time.

These changes are not dramatic in a few days. But over months and years, they make a remarkable difference.

Nutrition: The Foundation You Cannot Replace

Skin and hair depend on proper nutrition.

Hair is made largely of protein. Without enough protein, hair may become weak and thin.

Iron is essential for healthy hair growth. Low iron levels are a common cause of hair thinning, especially in women.

Vitamins support multiple functions. Vitamin C helps collagen formation. Vitamin D supports immune balance. B vitamins assist cell growth.

Healthy fats support the skin barrier, helping maintain softness and flexibility.

A balanced diet with whole foods is far more effective than relying on multiple supplements.

Doctor's Pearl

Supplements help only when there is a deficiency. They do not replace a balanced diet.

Hydration: Understanding the Reality

Water is important for overall health.

However, many people believe that drinking more water alone will cure dry skin.

In reality, dry skin is more often related to a damaged skin barrier than to dehydration.

Drinking adequate water is important, but applying moisturizer directly to the skin is often more effective for dryness.

Sleep: The Body's Repair Time

Sleep is when the body repairs itself.

During sleep, skin cells regenerate. Damage from daily exposure begins to heal.

Poor sleep can lead to dull skin, dark circles, and slower healing.

Chronic lack of sleep affects hormones and increases stress, which may worsen acne, hair shedding, and inflammatory conditions.

Sleep is not optional for healthy skin. It is essential.

Stress: The Silent Trigger

Stress affects the body in many ways.

It increases inflammation, alters hormones, and disrupts the hair growth cycle.

Many people notice increased hair shedding a few months after a stressful event.

Stress can also worsen acne, eczema, and psoriasis.

Managing stress does not mean eliminating it. It means responding to it in a healthier way.

Simple steps such as walking, maintaining routine, relaxation, and social connection can help.

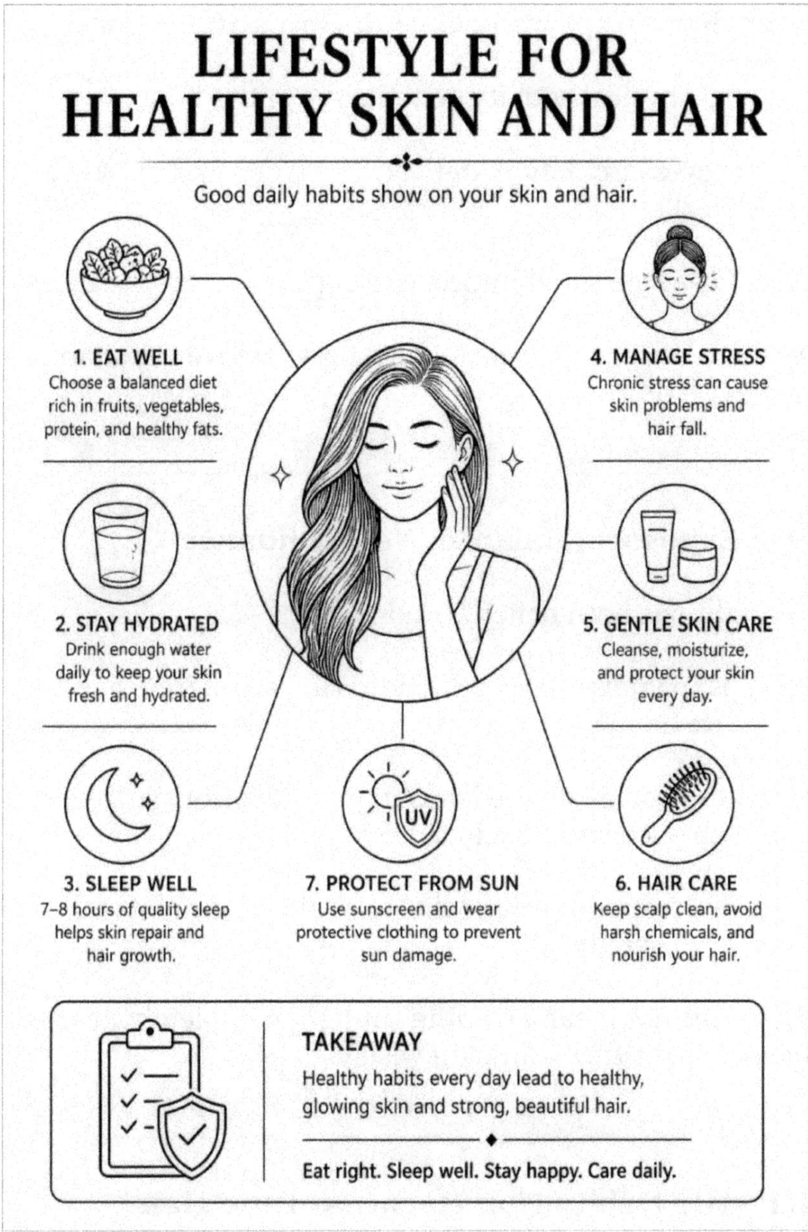
LIFESTYLE FOR HEALTHY SKIN AND HAIR
Good daily habits show on your skin and hair.
1. EAT WELL
Choose a balanced diet rich in fruits, vegetables, protein, and healthy fats.
4. MANAGE STRESS
Chronic stress can cause skin problems and hair fall.
2. STAY HYDRATED
Drink enough water daily to keep your skin fresh and hydrated.
5. GENTLE SKIN CARE
Cleanse, moisturize, and protect your skin every day.
UV
3. SLEEP WELL
7–8 hours of quality sleep helps skin repair and hair growth.
7. PROTECT FROM SUN
Use sunscreen and wear protective clothing to prevent sun damage.
6. HAIR CARE
Keep scalp clean, avoid harsh chemicals, and nourish your hair.
TAKEAWAY
Healthy habits every day lead to healthy, glowing skin and strong, beautiful hair.
Eat right. Sleep well. Stay happy. Care daily.

Exercise: Supporting Circulation and Balance

Regular physical activity benefits the entire body.

It improves circulation, delivering oxygen and nutrients to skin cells.

It reduces stress and improves sleep.

After exercise, gentle cleansing helps remove sweat and prevent irritation.

Sun Exposure: Balance, Not Avoidance

Sunlight has both benefits and risks.

It helps in vitamin D production. However, excessive exposure damages the skin.

Repeated sun exposure leads to pigmentation, wrinkles, and increased risk of skin cancer.

Daily protection is one of the most effective habits for long-term skin health.

This does not mean avoiding sunlight completely. It means protecting your skin wisely.

Lifestyle Habits That Harm Skin and Hair

Certain habits gradually damage skin and hair.

Smoking reduces blood flow and accelerates aging.

Excess alcohol affects hydration and skin quality.

Poor diet weakens overall health.

Irregular sleep and high stress increase inflammation.

Frequent use of harsh products damages the skin barrier.

These effects are gradual but significant.

Common Mistakes to Avoid

Relying only on supplements
Following extreme diets
Ignoring sleep
Underestimating stress
Expecting quick results

Myth vs Fact

Myth: Drinking large amounts of water cures dry skin.
Fact: Skin barrier care is more important.

Myth: Supplements replace a good diet.
Fact: They support only when needed.

Myth: Stress affects only the mind.
Fact: It affects skin and hair.

Myth: Exercise has no effect on skin.
Fact: It improves circulation and balance.

Red Flag Warnings

Seek medical advice if you notice:

- Hair loss with fatigue or poor nutrition
- Sudden weight loss with skin changes
- Severe sleep disturbance
- Persistent stress affecting daily life
- Signs of nutritional deficiency

Example: The Effect of Rapid Dieting

A 44-year-old woman follows a strict diet and loses weight quickly.

After a few months, she notices increased hair shedding.

The sudden dietary change disrupted her hair growth cycle.

With balanced nutrition and stabilization, her hair gradually improves.

Key Points

Lifestyle has a major impact on skin and hair.

Nutrition provides essential building blocks.

Sleep supports repair.

Stress affects hormones and inflammation.

Exercise improves circulation.

Chapter Summary

Healthy skin and hair are influenced by daily lifestyle choices. Nutrition, sleep, stress, and physical activity all play important roles.

Balanced habits are more effective than extreme measures.

Supplements have a limited role unless a deficiency exists.

Consistency in lifestyle leads to gradual and meaningful improvement.

Action Plan

• Maintain a balanced diet with adequate protein.

• Avoid extreme dieting.

• Stay reasonably hydrated.

- Prioritize regular sleep.
- Manage stress with simple habits.
- Exercise regularly.
- Protect your skin from excessive sun exposure.
- Be patient with results.

Bridge to the Next Chapter

Now that we understand the role of lifestyle, the next step is to apply this knowledge to daily skin care. In the next chapter, we will build a simple, effective routine that works in real life.

CHAPTER 9: Daily Skin Care Routine — Simple, Effective, and Realistic

Why Simple Wins Every Time

If there is one area where people feel overwhelmed, it is daily skin care.

Shelves are filled with cleansers, toners, serums, oils, masks, exfoliants, and creams. Each product promises better skin. Many routines suggest five, seven, or even ten steps.

In practice, most people do not need complicated routines.

In fact, the more complex the routine, the higher the chance of irritation, inconsistency, and confusion.

Healthy skin is usually maintained with a simple, steady approach.

The Three Essential Steps

For most people, a good skin care routine comes down to three core steps:

Cleansing
Moisturizing
Sun protection

Everything else is optional and depends on specific concerns.

If these three steps are done correctly and consistently, the skin often improves.

Cleansing: Clean Without Damaging

Cleansing removes dirt, sweat, oil, and environmental particles.

The goal is to clean the skin without stripping its natural protection.

Harsh soaps and strong cleansers can damage the skin barrier, leading to dryness and sensitivity.

A gentle cleanser is usually the best choice.

For oily skin, washing twice daily may help.
For dry or sensitive skin, once daily, usually at night, may be enough.

Water temperature matters. Lukewarm water is best. Hot water can damage the skin.

Doctor's Pearl

If your skin feels tight or uncomfortable after washing, your cleanser is too harsh.

Moisturizing: Supporting the Barrier

Moisturizers help retain water and support the skin barrier.

They reduce dryness, improve comfort, and protect against irritation.

Even oily skin benefits from a light moisturizer. Skipping it may lead to increased oil production.

Dry skin may need thicker creams. Oily skin may prefer lighter formulations.

Applying moisturizer soon after washing helps lock in moisture.

Sun Protection: The Most Important Habit

Sun exposure is a major cause of skin damage.

It contributes to pigmentation, wrinkles, uneven tone, and long-term risk of skin cancer.

Regular use of sunscreen is one of the most effective ways to protect the skin.

It should be applied to all exposed areas, including face, neck, and hands.

Protection is needed even on cloudy days.

Clothing, hats, and shade also provide protection.

Morning and Night Routine

A simple structure works best.

Morning

Gentle cleansing if needed
Moisturizer
Sunscreen

Night

Cleansing to remove dirt and oil
Moisturizer
Targeted treatment if needed

Optional Additions: Use Thoughtfully

Some products may be helpful for specific concerns.

Exfoliation may improve texture but should be gentle and limited.

Serums may help with acne, pigmentation, or aging.

Retinoids may be useful for certain conditions but require careful use.

The key is not to use everything at once.

DAILY SKIN & HAIR CARE ROUTINE

Simple steps every day for healthy skin and hair.

SKIN CARE ROUTINE

MORNING

1. CLEANSE
Wash your face gently to remove dirt and oil.

2. TREAT
Use a serum or treatment for your skin concern.

3. MOISTURIZE
Keep your skin hydrated and healthy.

4. PROTECT
Apply sunscreen to protect from sun damage.

EVENING

1. CLEANSE
Remove dirt, oil, and makeup.

2. TREAT
Use night serum or treatment.

3. MOISTURIZE
Replenish and repair your skin.

HAIR CARE ROUTINE

MORNING

1. BRUSH GENTLY
Brush your hair to remove tangles and stimulate scalp.

2. NOURISH
Apply light oil or serum to hair ends.

3. PROTECT
Protect hair from sun, heat, and pollution.

EVENING

1. CLEANSE (AS NEEDED)
Wash scalp with a mild shampoo.

2. CONDITION
Use conditioner to keep hair soft and smooth.

3. NOURISH
Apply oil to scalp or hair ends.

TAKEAWAY

Consistency is the key.
Small daily steps lead to healthy, glowing skin and strong, beautiful hair.

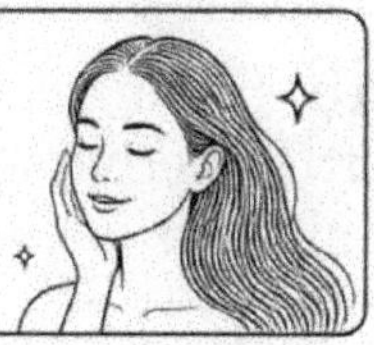

Understanding Your Skin Type

Skin care should match your skin type.

Dry skin feels rough and tight and needs more hydration.

Oily skin appears shiny and may need lighter products.

Combination skin has both dry and oily areas.

Sensitive skin reacts easily and needs gentle care.

Skin type may change with age, weather, and health.

Common Mistakes to Avoid

Using too many products
Changing products frequently
Over-exfoliating
Using harsh scrubs
Skipping sunscreen
Expecting quick results

Myth vs Fact

Myth: Expensive products work better.
Fact: Effectiveness depends on ingredients and suitability.

Myth: Natural products are always safe.
Fact: They can also irritate.

Myth: Scrubbing improves skin.
Fact: It damages the barrier.

Myth: More products give better results.
Fact: Simplicity often works best.

Red Flag Warnings

Seek medical advice if you notice:

- Persistent irritation
- Burning or peeling
- Worsening acne or rash
- Allergic reactions
- No improvement despite consistent care

Example: The Overloaded Routine

A 45-year-old woman uses multiple products daily, including exfoliants and serums.

Her skin becomes red and sensitive.

When she reduces her routine to cleansing, moisturizing, and sun protection, her skin improves.

This illustrates the power of simplicity.

Key Points

Simple routines are effective.

Cleansing, moisturizing, and sun protection are essential.

Overuse of products can damage the skin.

Skin type should guide choices.

Consistency matters more than complexity.

Chapter Summary

Daily skin care does not need to be complicated. A gentle cleanser, a suitable moisturizer, and regular sun protection form the foundation of healthy skin.

Additional products may be useful for specific concerns but should be used carefully.

Consistency and simplicity lead to better long-term results.

Action Plan

- Use a gentle cleanser once or twice daily.
- Apply moisturizer suited to your skin type.
- Use sunscreen regularly.
- Avoid adding multiple new products at once.

- Introduce active ingredients slowly.
- Stop products that irritate your skin.
- Keep your routine simple and consistent.
- Be patient with results.

Bridge to the Next Chapter

Now that we have built a simple daily routine, the next step is to understand what is inside these products. In the next chapter, we will break down key ingredients, what truly works, and how to avoid confusion.

CHAPTER 10: Understanding Products and Ingredients — What Works, What Doesn't, and What to Avoid

From Labels to Logic

Most confusion in skin and hair care begins with product labels.

Long ingredient lists, scientific names, bold claims, and persuasive marketing can make everything sound important.

But here is the truth.

You do not need to understand every ingredient. You need to understand the few that matter.

Once you learn how to think about ingredients, your choices become clearer, simpler, and more effective.

Start with a Simple Principle

A few well-chosen ingredients, used consistently, work better than many used without understanding.

Doctor's Pearl

Do not build your routine around products. Build it around your skin problem.

Key Ingredients That Truly Help

Let us focus on ingredients with strong evidence and practical value.

Retinoids (Vitamin A Derivatives)
These are among the most studied ingredients.

They help improve acne, support skin renewal, and reduce fine lines over time.

They can be effective, but may cause dryness or irritation when first used. They should be introduced gradually.

Vitamin C
This is an antioxidant.

It helps reduce pigmentation, supports collagen formation, and protects against environmental damage.

Results are gradual, and stability of the product matters.

Niacinamide (Vitamin B3)
A versatile and well-tolerated ingredient.

It supports the skin barrier, reduces redness, and helps balance oil production.

Suitable for most skin types.

Hyaluronic Acid
This helps retain moisture.

It improves hydration and gives a temporary plumping effect.

Works best when combined with a moisturizer.

Ceramides
These are natural components of the skin barrier.

They help repair and maintain the barrier.

Especially useful for dry and sensitive skin.

Salicylic Acid
Useful for acne.

It helps clear pores and reduce inflammation.

Excessive use may cause dryness.

Benzoyl Peroxide
Helps reduce bacteria involved in acne.

Effective but may cause dryness or irritation.

Should be used carefully.

Sunscreen Ingredients
Essential for protecting the skin from ultraviolet damage.

They help prevent pigmentation, premature aging, and skin cancer.

Daily use is one of the most important steps in skin care.

Hair Care Ingredients That Matter

Hair care is often overcomplicated.

A few ingredients are truly useful.

Minoxidil
Widely used for certain types of hair loss.

It helps stimulate hair growth and slow hair thinning.

Requires consistent, long-term use.

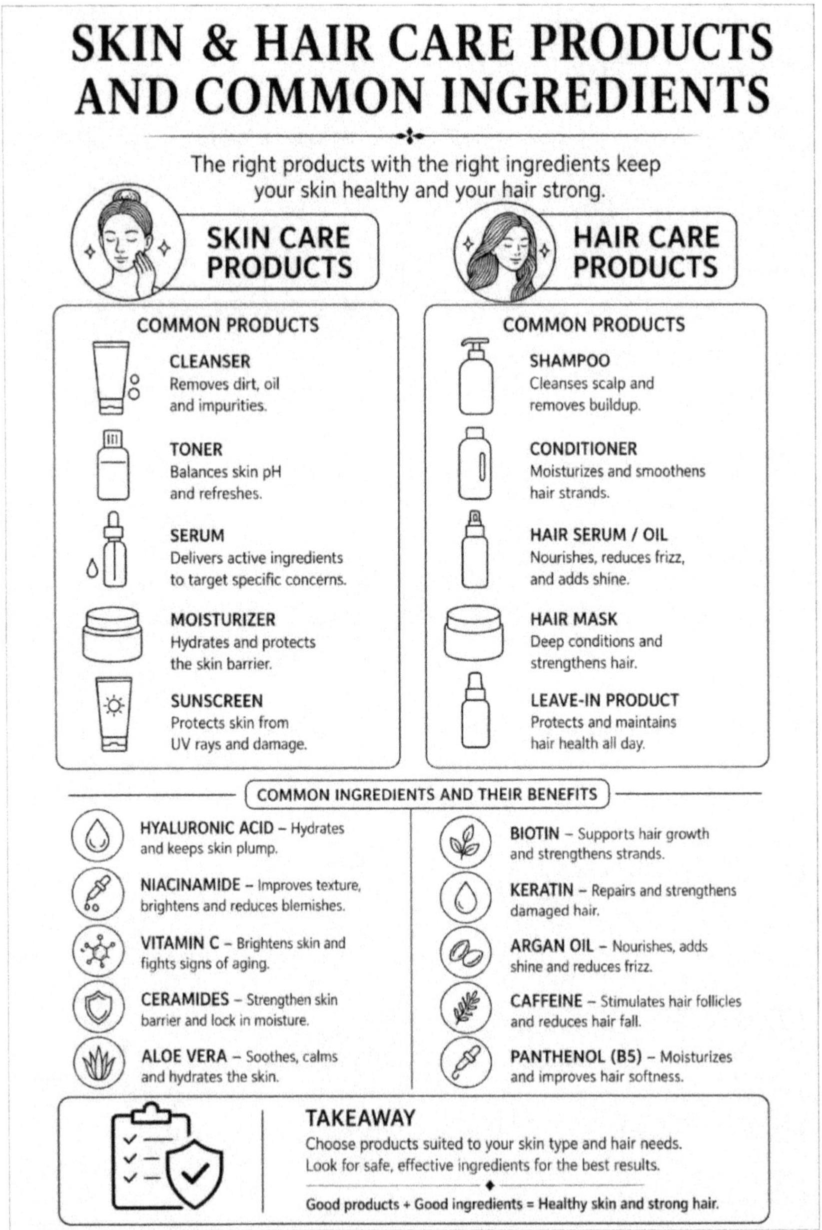
SKIN & HAIR CARE PRODUCTS AND COMMON INGREDIENTS
The right products with the right ingredients keep your skin healthy and your hair strong.
SKIN CARE PRODUCTS
COMMON PRODUCTS
CLEANSER
Removes dirt, oil and impurities.
TONER
Balances skin pH and refreshes.
SERUM
Delivers active ingredients to target specific concerns.
MOISTURIZER
Hydrates and protects the skin barrier.
SUNSCREEN
Protects skin from UV rays and damage.
HAIR CARE PRODUCTS
COMMON PRODUCTS
SHAMPOO
Cleanses scalp and removes buildup.
CONDITIONER
Moisturizes and smoothens hair strands.
HAIR SERUM / OIL
Nourishes, reduces frizz, and adds shine.
HAIR MASK
Deep conditions and strengthens hair.
LEAVE-IN PRODUCT
Protects and maintains hair health all day.
COMMON INGREDIENTS AND THEIR BENEFITS
HYALURONIC ACID – Hydrates and keeps skin plump.
NIACINAMIDE – Improves texture, brightens and reduces blemishes.
VITAMIN C – Brightens skin and fights signs of aging.
CERAMIDES – Strengthen skin barrier and lock in moisture.
ALOE VERA – Soothes, calms and hydrates the skin.
BIOTIN – Supports hair growth and strengthens strands.
KERATIN – Repairs and strengthens damaged hair.
ARGAN OIL – Nourishes, adds shine and reduces frizz.
CAFFEINE – Stimulates hair follicles and reduces hair fall.
PANTHENOL (B5) – Moisturizes and improves hair softness.
TAKEAWAY
Choose products suited to your skin type and hair needs.
Look for safe, effective ingredients for the best results.
Good products + Good ingredients = Healthy skin and strong hair.

Ketoconazole (in shampoos)
Useful for dandruff and certain scalp conditions.

Helps reduce inflammation and fungal growth.

Conditioning Agents
Improve hair softness and reduce breakage.

They improve appearance but do not treat hair loss.

Biotin and Hair Supplements

Biotin is often promoted for hair growth.

It helps mainly when there is a deficiency, which is uncommon.

Most people do not benefit significantly from supplements without a clear deficiency.

"Natural" vs "Chemical": A Misleading Debate

Many products are labeled as "natural" or "chemical-free."

This can be confusing.

Everything, including natural substances, is made of chemicals.

Natural ingredients can also cause irritation or allergy.

Safety depends on formulation, not the label.

How to Read Labels Without Stress

You do not need to analyze every ingredient.

Focus on:

The main active ingredient
Whether it matches your concern
Whether the product suits your skin type

Avoid products with unnecessary additives, especially if you have sensitive skin.

Common Ingredient Mistakes

Using multiple active ingredients together
Starting strong products too quickly
Mixing incompatible treatments
Expecting immediate results
Stopping too early

These mistakes often lead to irritation or poor results.

Myth vs Fact

Myth: More active ingredients mean better results.
Fact: Too many can irritate the skin.

Myth: Natural products are always safer.
Fact: They can also cause reactions.

Myth: Expensive products are more effective.
Fact: Effectiveness depends on ingredients.

Myth: Supplements replace proper care.
Fact: They have a limited role.

Red Flag Warnings

Be cautious if you notice:

- Burning or stinging
- Severe irritation
- Sudden worsening of symptoms
- Allergic reactions
- No improvement despite use

Example: Too Many Actives

A 44-year-old man starts using multiple products containing retinoids, acids, and vitamin C together.

His skin becomes irritated within days.

When he simplifies his routine and introduces one product at a time, his skin improves.

This highlights the importance of a structured approach.

Key Points

A few well-chosen ingredients are enough.

Retinoids, niacinamide, and sunscreen are widely useful.

Minoxidil helps certain types of hair loss.

Supplements help only when deficiency exists.

Simple routines work best.

Chapter Summary

Understanding ingredients allows you to make informed decisions and avoid confusion. Some ingredients have strong scientific support and are widely useful, while others are helpful only in specific situations.

Many products are over-marketed.

A simple, targeted approach using the right ingredients leads to better outcomes.

Action Plan

- Identify your main concern before choosing products.

- Use a few well-chosen ingredients.
- Introduce new products one at a time.
- Avoid combining multiple strong ingredients.
- Do not rely on marketing claims.
- Be patient and consistent.
- Seek guidance if needed.

Bridge to the Next Chapter

Now that you understand ingredients, the next step is to apply this knowledge to real conditions. In the next chapter, we will begin with one of the most common problems: acne, and how to manage it effectively.

CHAPTER 11: Acne — From Teenage Breakouts to Adult Struggles

A Condition Almost Everyone Encounters

Acne is one of the most common skin conditions I see in practice.

It does not belong only to teenagers. It often begins in adolescence, but it may continue into adulthood or even appear for the first time later in life.

For some, it is mild and occasional. For others, it becomes persistent, painful, and emotionally distressing.

Acne is not just about appearance. It can affect confidence, social interaction, and quality of life. When not treated properly, it can leave lasting marks.

The encouraging part is this. Acne is manageable. But it requires understanding, patience, and the right approach.

What Really Causes Acne

Acne develops due to a combination of factors working together.

The skin contains oil glands that produce sebum. In some individuals, these glands are more active.

Excess oil mixes with dead skin cells and blocks pores.

Bacteria that normally live on the skin multiply within these blocked pores.

This leads to inflammation.

Hormones play a central role. They increase oil production, which is why acne often begins during puberty. Hormonal fluctuations can also trigger acne in adults, especially in women.

Genetics also influence how prone a person is to acne.

Doctor's Pearl

Acne is not caused by dirty skin. Over-washing often makes it worse.

Types of Acne

Acne does not look the same in everyone.

Whiteheads and blackheads are non-inflammatory.

Papules and pustules are inflamed.

Nodules and cysts are deeper and more severe. These are more likely to cause scarring.

Recognizing the type helps guide treatment.

DRY SKIN, ECZEMA & ALLERGIC REACTIONS

Know the difference. Care the right way.

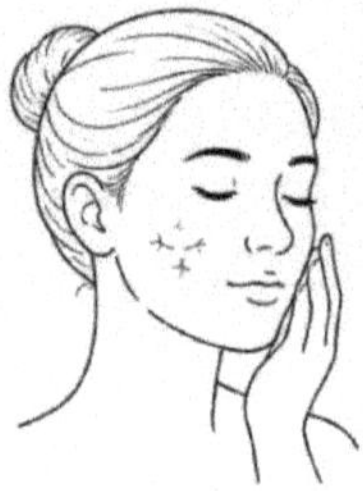

DRY SKIN

Lack of moisture makes the skin rough, flaky or tight.

COMMON SIGNS

- Rough, flaky skin
- Tightness, especially after washing
- Itching

COMMON CAUSES

- Cold, dry weather
- Hot showers, harsh soaps
- Low humidity

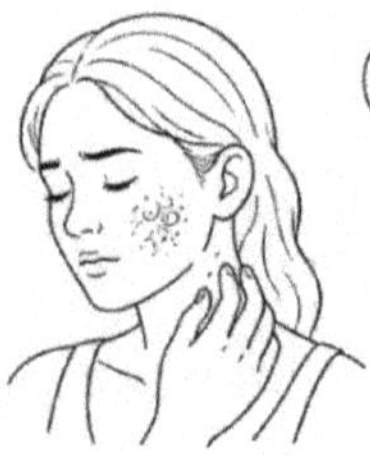

ECZEMA

A chronic condition that causes inflamed, itchy and irritated skin.

COMMON SIGNS

- Red, inflamed patches
- Itching (worse at night)
- Dry, scaly or thickened skin

COMMON TRIGGERS

- Irritants (soaps, detergents)
- Allergens (dust, pollen)
- Stress

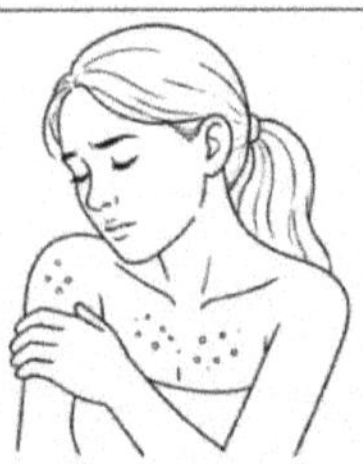

ALLERGIC REACTIONS

The skin reacts to an allergen causing redness, itching or rashes.

COMMON SIGNS

- Redness or hives
- Itching or burning
- Rashes or bumps

COMMON CAUSES

- Cosmetics, perfumes
- Certain foods
- Medications, insect bites

SIMPLE CARE TIPS (FOR ALL THREE)

- Use gentle cleansers
- Moisturize regularly
- Stay hydrated (drink water)
- Protect skin from sun and harsh weather

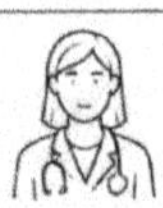

WHEN TO SEE A DOCTOR?

- Symptoms are severe or worsening
- No improvement with self-care
- Skin is cracked, oozing or infected

TAKEAWAY

Understand your skin.
Treat gently. Stay consistent.
Healthy skin, happy you.

Teenage Acne vs Adult Acne

Teenage acne usually affects the forehead, nose, and cheeks. It is mainly related to increased oil production.

Adult acne often appears along the jawline, chin, and neck. Hormonal influence is stronger.

Adult acne may also occur along with sensitive or aging skin, which makes treatment more delicate.

What Makes Acne Worse

Certain factors can aggravate acne.

Hormonal fluctuations
Stress
Certain cosmetics or skin care products
Heavy or oily products
Friction from masks or clothing
Certain medications

Diet may influence acne in some individuals, though the effect varies.

Skin Care for Acne-Prone Skin

A simple routine works best.

Use a gentle cleanser.
Avoid harsh scrubbing.

Use non-comedogenic products.
Apply a light moisturizer if needed.

Overloading the skin with multiple products often worsens acne.

Doctor's Pearl

Irritated skin breaks out more easily. Keep your routine calm and simple.

Basic Treatments That Help

Mild acne may improve with simple treatments.

Salicylic acid helps unclog pores.

Benzoyl peroxide reduces bacteria and inflammation.

These should be used carefully to avoid irritation.

Improvement takes time.

When Medical Treatment Is Needed

Moderate to severe acne often requires medical treatment.

Topical retinoids help prevent blocked pores.

Antibiotics may be used for inflammation.

Hormonal treatment may help selected patients.

Stronger medications may be needed for severe cases.

Treatment must be individualized.

Scars and Marks: Why Early Care Matters

One of the biggest concerns with acne is scarring.

Picking or squeezing pimples increases the risk.

Inflammatory acne is more likely to leave marks.

Once scars develop, they are difficult to treat.

Early treatment helps prevent long-term damage.

Common Mistakes to Avoid

Washing the face too frequently
Using harsh scrubs
Popping pimples
Using too many products
Stopping treatment too early

Myth vs Fact

Myth: Acne is caused by dirty skin.
Fact: It is caused by oil, bacteria, and inflammation.

Myth: Sun exposure cures acne.
Fact: It may worsen long-term damage.

Myth: Only teenagers get acne.
Fact: Adults commonly have acne.

Myth: Home remedies always help.
Fact: Some may irritate the skin.

Red Flag Warnings

Seek medical advice if you notice:

- Severe or painful acne
- Acne that does not improve
- Acne causing scars
- Sudden severe acne
- Acne with hormonal symptoms

Example: Hormonal Acne in Adulthood

A 35-year-old woman develops persistent acne along the jawline. She tries multiple products without improvement.

Evaluation shows a hormonal pattern.

With appropriate treatment, her acne improves gradually.

This highlights the importance of identifying the cause.

Key Points

Acne is common and manageable.

It results from multiple factors.

Different types need different treatments.

Early treatment helps prevent scarring.

Simple routines work best.

Chapter Summary

Acne is a multifactorial condition influenced by oil production, blocked pores, bacteria, and inflammation. It affects both teenagers and adults.

Mild acne may respond to simple care, while more severe forms require medical treatment.

Early and consistent treatment helps prevent scarring and long-term problems.

Action Plan

- Identify your acne type.
- Use a gentle cleansing routine.
- Start simple treatments and use them consistently.
- Avoid picking or squeezing lesions.
- Watch for triggers.
- Seek medical care if acne is severe or persistent.
- Be patient. Improvement takes time.

Bridge to the Next Chapter

Acne is common, but many people struggle with dryness, itching, and allergic reactions. In the next chapter, we will explore eczema, dry skin, and skin allergies, and how to manage them effectively.

CHAPTER 12: Dry Skin, Eczema, and Allergic Reactions — Breaking the Itch Cycle

When Comfort Disappears

For many people, skin problems do not begin with what they see. They begin with what they feel.

A tight sensation after washing.
An itch that worsens at night.
Skin that feels rough, sensitive, or easily irritated.

At first, it may seem minor. Over time, it can become constant.

Dry skin, eczema, and allergic reactions are among the most common reasons people feel uncomfortable in their own skin. They can affect sleep, concentration, and daily life.

The good news is that these conditions are usually manageable when you understand the underlying problem.

Dry Skin: A Barrier Problem, Not Just Lack of Water

Dry skin is often misunderstood.

It is not simply due to not drinking enough water. The main issue is the skin barrier.

When the barrier is weak, the skin cannot retain moisture. Water escapes, and irritants enter.

This leads to:

Dryness
Roughness
Sensitivity
Mild itching

Common causes include:

Aging
Cold or dry weather
Hot showers
Harsh soaps
Frequent washing

Doctor's Pearl

Treat dryness by repairing the skin barrier, not by over-washing or scrubbing.

Eczema: More Than Just Dry Skin

Eczema, also called atopic dermatitis, is a common condition.

It causes:

Intense itching
Red or darker patches
Dry, rough skin
Thickening from repeated scratching

It often affects the face, neck, hands, and skin folds such as elbows and knees.

Eczema is influenced by genetics, environment, and immune response.

It tends to flare and improve in cycles.

Triggers That Worsen Eczema

Certain factors commonly trigger flare-ups.

Harsh soaps and detergents
Fragrances and cosmetics
Rough fabrics such as wool
Stress
Weather changes
Sweating

Identifying triggers is a key part of long-term control.

The Itch-Scratch Cycle

One of the most important concepts in eczema is the itch-scratch cycle.

The skin itches.
You scratch.
The skin becomes damaged.
Inflammation increases.
The itching worsens.

This cycle continues unless it is interrupted.

Doctor's Pearl

Relieving itching is not only about comfort. It prevents further skin damage.

Contact Dermatitis: Reaction to Something You Touch

Contact dermatitis occurs when the skin reacts to an external substance.

This may be due to:

Irritants such as detergents or chemicals
Allergens such as fragrances, metals, or cosmetics

The rash usually appears at the site of contact.

It may be red, itchy, swollen, or blistering.

Avoiding the trigger is the most important step in treatment.

Allergic Reactions: From Mild to Severe

Allergic reactions vary in severity.

Mild reactions may cause itching and rash.

Severe reactions may include swelling of the face or lips, or difficulty breathing.

Severe reactions require immediate medical attention.

Repeated mild reactions should be evaluated to identify the cause.

Daily Care That Makes a Difference

Simple habits can greatly improve dry and sensitive skin.

Use gentle, fragrance-free cleansers
Avoid long, hot showers
Pat the skin dry, do not rub
Apply moisturizer immediately after bathing
Wear soft, breathable fabrics
Keep nails short to reduce damage from scratching

Consistency is more important than intensity.

DRY SKIN, ECZEMA & ALLERGIC REACTIONS

Know the difference. Care the right way.

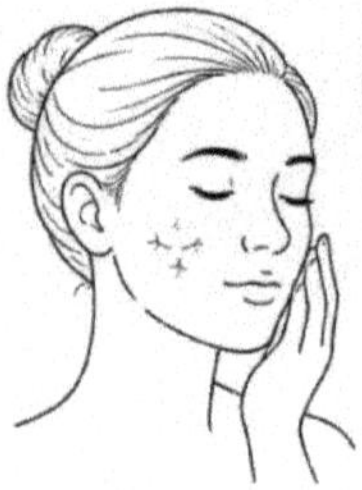

DRY SKIN

Lack of moisture makes the skin rough, flaky or tight.

COMMON SIGNS

- Rough, flaky skin
- Tightness, especially after washing
- Itching

COMMON CAUSES

- Cold, dry weather
- Hot showers, harsh soaps
- Low humidity

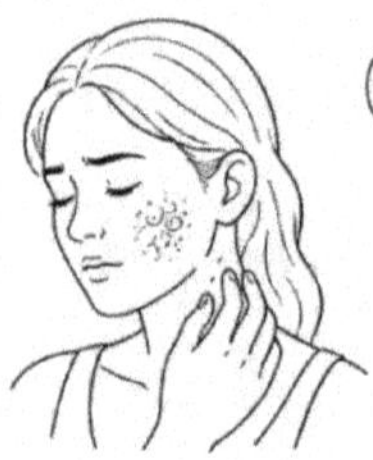

ECZEMA

A chronic condition that causes inflamed, itchy and irritated skin.

COMMON SIGNS

- Red, inflamed patches
- Itching (worse at night)
- Dry, scaly or thickened skin

COMMON TRIGGERS

- Irritants (soaps, detergents)
- Allergens (dust, pollen)
- Stress

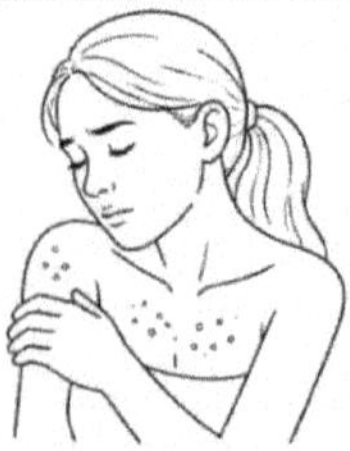

ALLERGIC REACTIONS

The skin reacts to an allergen causing redness, itching or rashes.

COMMON SIGNS

- Redness or hives
- Itching or burning
- Rashes or bumps

COMMON CAUSES

- Cosmetics, perfumes
- Certain foods
- Medications, insect bites

SIMPLE CARE TIPS (FOR ALL THREE)

- Use gentle cleansers
- Moisturize regularly
- Stay hydrated (drink water)
- Protect skin from sun and harsh weather

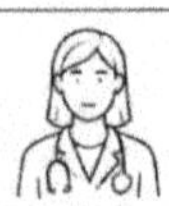

WHEN TO SEE A DOCTOR?

- Symptoms are severe or worsening
- No improvement with self-care
- Skin is cracked, oozing or infected

TAKEAWAY

Understand your skin.
Treat gently. Stay consistent.
Healthy skin, happy you.

Treatment Approach

Management depends on severity.

Moisturizing is the foundation.

Avoiding triggers prevents flare-ups.

Medications may be needed during flare-ups to reduce inflammation.

Severe or persistent cases require medical care.

Common Mistakes to Avoid

Using harsh soaps or scrubs
Taking very hot showers
Ignoring persistent itching
Using multiple products without understanding
Scratching repeatedly
Stopping treatment too early

Myth vs Fact

Myth: Dry skin is due only to lack of water intake.
Fact: The skin barrier plays the main role.

Myth: Eczema is contagious.
Fact: It is not.

Myth: Scratching helps relieve itching.
Fact: It worsens the condition over time.

Myth: All rashes are allergies.
Fact: Many have different causes.

Red Flag Warnings

Seek medical advice if you notice:

- Severe or persistent itching
- Rapidly spreading rash
- Signs of infection such as pain, swelling, or pus
- Swelling of face or lips
- Difficulty breathing with rash
- Skin that becomes thick or discolored

Example: The Fragrance Trigger

A 47-year-old man develops an itchy rash on his neck after using a new perfume.

He continues using it, assuming the skin will adjust.

The rash worsens.

When he stops the product and receives proper treatment, the skin improves.

This highlights the importance of identifying triggers early.

Key Points

Dry skin is mainly due to barrier dysfunction.

Eczema causes chronic itching and inflammation.

Contact dermatitis results from exposure to irritants or allergens.

Scratching worsens the condition.

Simple, consistent care is effective.

Chapter Summary

Dry skin, eczema, and allergic reactions are common conditions that affect comfort and quality of life. They are usually related to barrier dysfunction, environmental triggers, and immune response.

Understanding the cause, avoiding triggers, and maintaining gentle skin care are essential for long-term control.

Breaking the itch-scratch cycle is a key part of treatment.

Action Plan

- Use gentle, fragrance-free products.

- Moisturize regularly.
- Avoid hot showers and harsh scrubbing.
- Identify and avoid triggers.
- Keep nails short.
- Seek medical care for persistent symptoms.
- Follow treatment consistently.

Bridge to the Next Chapter

While dryness and allergies are common, some skin conditions are more chronic and persistent. In the next chapter, we will explore psoriasis, rosacea, and other long-term inflammatory conditions, and how to manage them effectively.

CHAPTER 13: Psoriasis, Rosacea, and Chronic Skin Conditions — Learning Long-Term Control

When Skin Problems Do Not Fully Go Away

Some skin conditions behave differently.

They do not disappear completely.
They improve, then return.
They flare, then settle, then flare again.

This pattern can be frustrating. Many people try treatment after treatment, hoping for a permanent cure.

The truth is important to understand.

Some skin conditions are chronic. They are controlled, not cured.

Once you accept this, your approach becomes calmer, more practical, and more effective.

Psoriasis: A Condition Beneath the Surface

Psoriasis is not just a surface rash.

It is an inflammatory condition involving the immune system.

The skin produces new cells faster than normal. These cells accumulate, forming thick, scaly patches.

Common sites include:

Elbows
Knees
Scalp
Lower back

The patches may be itchy, dry, or uncomfortable.

In lighter skin, they appear red with silvery scales. In darker skin, they may appear darker or purplish.

Doctor's Pearl

Psoriasis is not contagious. It is a chronic inflammatory condition that can be controlled.

Psoriasis and Joint Symptoms

Some people with psoriasis develop joint problems.

This is called psoriatic arthritis.

Symptoms may include:

Joint pain
Stiffness
Swelling

Early recognition is important because untreated joint inflammation can lead to long-term damage.

Triggers That Cause Flare-Ups

Psoriasis often follows a pattern of flares.

Common triggers include:

Stress
Infections
Skin injury
Certain medications
Cold weather

Understanding personal triggers helps reduce flare-ups.

Rosacea: Sensitive Skin with Persistent Redness

Rosacea mainly affects the face.

It often begins with flushing, which gradually becomes persistent redness.

Other features may include:

Small bumps
Visible blood vessels
Burning or stinging
Sensitive skin

It is often mistaken for acne, but the cause and treatment are different.

Common Rosacea Triggers

Sun exposure
Hot beverages
Spicy food
Alcohol
Stress
Temperature changes

Avoiding triggers is a key part of management.

Doctor's Pearl

If your skin reacts easily, simplify your routine before adding more treatment.

Chronic Sensitive Skin

Some individuals have skin that reacts to multiple products or environmental changes.

This may not fit into a single diagnosis but reflects a sensitive skin pattern.

In such cases, a simple routine with minimal products is often the best approach.

PSORIASIS, ROSACEA & CHRONIC SKIN CONDITIONS

Understand. Identify. Care.

PSORIASIS

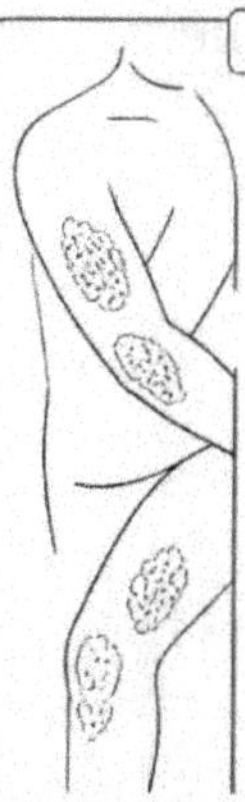

A chronic autoimmune condition that speeds up skin cell growth, causing scales and inflammation.

COMMON SIGNS

- Red, raised patches
- Silvery-white scales
- Itching, burning or soreness
- Dry, cracked skin

COMMON TRIGGERS

- Stress
- Infections
- Cold, dry weather
- Certain medications

ROSACEA

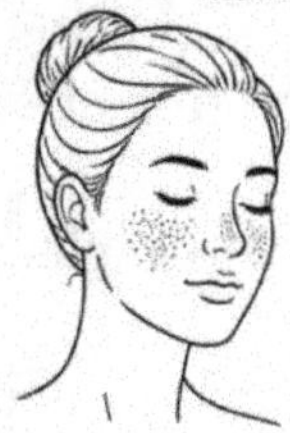

A chronic condition that causes redness and visible blood vessels, mainly on the face.

COMMON SIGNS

- Facial redness
- Visible blood vessels
- Bumps or pimples
- Burning or stinging

COMMON TRIGGERS

- Sun exposure
- Spicy food & hot drinks
- Alcohol
- Stress, extreme temperatures

OTHER CHRONIC SKIN CONDITIONS

ATOPIC DERMATITIS (ECZEMA)

Causes dry, itchy, inflamed skin. Often linked to allergies and family history.

- Dry, scaly patches
- Intense itching
- Flare-ups come and go

VITILIGO

Loss of skin color in patches due to reduced melanin.

- White patches on skin
- Common on face, hands, elbows, knees
- Not contagious

LUPUS (CUTANEOUS)

Autoimmune condition that can cause rashes, lesions or sensitivity to sunlight.

- Red, scaly patches
- Butterfly rash on face
- Fatigue, joint pain may occur

GENERAL CARE TIPS (HELPFUL FOR ALL)

- Use gentle, fragrance-free skincare
- Moisturize daily
- Protect skin from the sun (SPF 30+)
- Stay hydrated and eat a balanced diet
- Manage stress and get enough sleep
- Follow medical advice and treatment

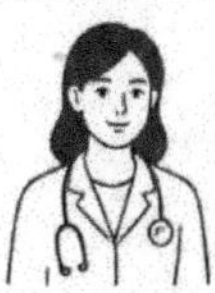

WHEN TO SEE A DOCTOR?

- Symptoms are severe or persistent
- Affecting daily life or confidence
- Not improving with self-care
- Signs of infection (oozing, pus, increased pain)

TAKEAWAY

These conditions are chronic, but manageable. With the right care, lifestyle and treatment, you can live a healthy, confident and comfortable life.

Your skin is unique. Be kind to it. Consistent care makes a big difference.

The Emotional Impact

Chronic skin conditions can affect confidence.

Visible skin changes may lead to self-consciousness.

Unpredictable flare-ups create frustration.

It is important to acknowledge these effects.

Managing these conditions improves both physical comfort and emotional well-being.

Treatment Approach: Control, Not Cure

Treatment aims to reduce symptoms and prevent flare-ups.

Options may include:

Topical medications
Oral medications in selected cases
Lifestyle adjustments
Trigger avoidance

Consistency is essential.

Stopping treatment too early often leads to recurrence.

Common Mistakes to Avoid

Expecting a permanent cure
Stopping treatment once symptoms improve
Using harsh or irritating products
Ignoring triggers
Self-treating without proper diagnosis

Myth vs Fact

Myth: Psoriasis is an infection.
Fact: It is an immune-related condition.

Myth: Rosacea is the same as acne.
Fact: They are different conditions.

Myth: Chronic skin problems can be cured permanently.
Fact: They are usually managed.

Myth: If symptoms improve, treatment can stop completely.
Fact: Maintenance is often needed.

Red Flag Warnings

Seek medical advice if you notice:

- Severe or widespread skin lesions
- Joint pain with skin symptoms
- Persistent facial redness with discomfort
- Thickening or deformity of skin
- No improvement with basic care

Example: Recognizing a Pattern

A 52-year-old woman experiences repeated facial redness. She notices it worsens after hot drinks and stress.

By identifying these triggers and simplifying her routine, she gains better control of her symptoms.

This shows the importance of observing patterns.

Key Points

Chronic skin conditions are long-term but manageable.

Psoriasis involves inflammation and rapid skin growth.

Rosacea causes facial redness and sensitivity.

Triggers play a major role.

Consistency is essential.

Chapter Summary

Chronic skin conditions such as psoriasis and rosacea behave differently from short-term problems. They involve ongoing inflammation and are influenced by triggers and individual sensitivity.

While they may not be completely cured, they can be effectively controlled.

Understanding triggers, using appropriate treatment, and maintaining consistency lead to better outcomes.

Action Plan

- Identify your personal triggers.
- Keep a simple record of flare patterns.
- Use gentle skin care.
- Follow treatment consistently.
- Avoid stopping treatment suddenly.
- Seek medical advice when needed.
- Focus on long-term control.

Bridge to the Next Chapter

Chronic conditions are important, but infections are also very common and often confused with other problems. In the next chapter, we will explore bacterial, fungal, and viral skin infections, and how to recognize and treat them correctly.

CHAPTER 14: Skin Infections – Recognizing Them Early and Treating Them Right

When the Skin Barrier Is Breached

Your skin does a remarkable job protecting you every day.

It acts as a shield against bacteria, fungi, and viruses that are constantly present in the environment. Most of the time, this protection works silently and effectively.

But when the barrier is disrupted, even slightly, germs find an opportunity.

A small cut. Repeated scratching. Excess moisture in skin folds. An underlying skin condition.

These are enough to allow infection to develop.

Skin infections are common. They are also frequently misunderstood, which leads to delayed or incorrect treatment.

Why Infections Are Often Missed

Many infections look similar to other skin conditions.

A fungal infection may resemble eczema.
A bacterial infection may look like simple irritation.
A viral rash may be mistaken for an allergy.

This confusion often leads to the use of the wrong treatment.

Instead of improving, the condition spreads or becomes persistent.

Recognizing patterns early makes a significant difference.

Doctor's Pearl

If a rash is spreading or not improving with simple care, reconsider the diagnosis.

Bacterial Infections: When Pain and Warmth Are Clues

Bacterial infections often begin where the skin is broken.

Common features include:

Redness
Warmth
Swelling
Pain
Sometimes pus or discharge

The affected area may feel tender and may enlarge over time.

In some cases, a localized collection of pus may form. In others, the infection may spread over a wider area.

If untreated, bacterial infections can progress.

Fungal Infections: Common but Often Misdiagnosed

Fungal infections thrive in warm, moist areas.

They often appear as:

Itchy, red or darker patches
Clear or well-defined borders
Scaling
Sometimes a ring-like pattern

Common areas include:

Feet
Groin
Underarms
Body folds
Scalp

A common mistake is treating fungal infections with creams meant for other conditions. This may reduce redness temporarily but allows the infection to persist or spread.

Yeast Infections of the Skin

Yeast is a type of fungus.

It commonly affects areas where moisture is trapped.

Features include:

Redness
Irritation
Itching
Small surrounding spots

These infections are more common in people with diabetes, those who sweat heavily, or in areas with poor ventilation.

Keeping the area dry is an important part of treatment.

Viral Infections: Different Patterns

Viral infections can present in different ways.

Cold sores appear as painful blisters near the lips.

Warts appear as small growths on the skin.

Shingles presents as a painful rash, usually on one side of the body.

Some viral infections resolve on their own. Others require treatment.

Shingles: Recognize It Early

Shingles often begins with pain, burning, or tingling before a rash appears.

The rash usually follows a specific pattern on one side of the body.

Early treatment can reduce severity and complications.

Vaccination is available and can reduce risk in appropriate individuals.

Why Correct Diagnosis Matters

Using the wrong treatment delays recovery.

A fungal infection treated as eczema may worsen.

A bacterial infection ignored may spread.

A viral condition may need timely treatment to prevent complications.

When in doubt, proper evaluation is essential.

Common Mistakes to Avoid

Using random creams
Stopping treatment too early
Ignoring spreading rash
Sharing personal items such as towels
Keeping infected areas moist

COMMON SKIN INFECTIONS

Know the signs. Get the right care.

1. FUNGAL INFECTIONS (Ringworm)

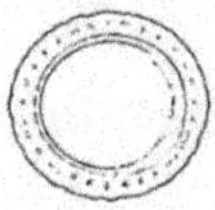

Caused by fungi (ringworm) that grow on the skin.

COMMON SIGNS
- Itchy, red, ring-shaped rash
- Scaly or flaky skin
- May spread slowly

CAUSE
Fungi; spreads by direct contact or sharing items.

2. BACTERIAL INFECTIONS (Impetigo)

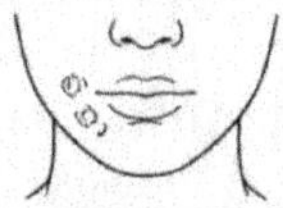

Caused by bacteria entering the skin through cuts or sores.

COMMON SIGNS
- Red sores or blisters
- Honey-colored crusts
- Pain or tenderness

CAUSE
Bacteria (Staphylococcus or Streptococcus).

3. VIRAL INFECTIONS (Herpes Simplex)

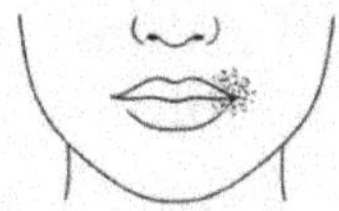

Caused by a virus that affects the skin and nerves.

COMMON SIGNS
- Painful blisters or bumps
- Itching or tingling
- Crusting and healing

CAUSE
Herpes simplex virus (HSV-1 commonly causes cold sores).

4. YEAST INFECTIONS (Candidiasis)

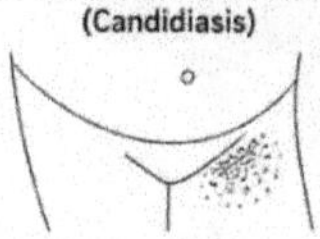

Caused by excess growth of yeast (Candida) on the skin.

COMMON SIGNS
- Red, itchy rash
- Burning or soreness
- Often occurs in skin folds

CAUSE
Yeast overgrowth; moisture, heat, poor hygiene.

5. SCABIES

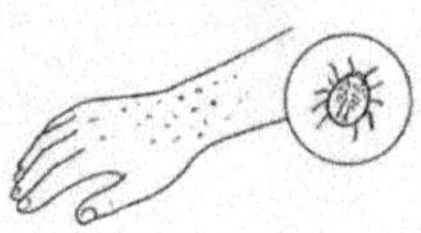

Caused by tiny mites that burrow into the skin.

COMMON SIGNS
- Intense itching (worse at night)
- Small red bumps or blisters
- Burrows or sores

CAUSE
Sarcoptes scabiei mite; spreads by close contact.

6. CELLULITIS

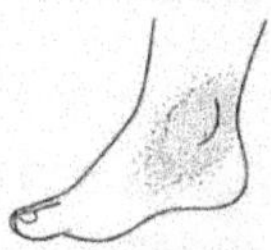

A bacterial infection of deeper layers of the skin.

COMMON SIGNS
- Red, swollen, warm skin
- Pain or tenderness
- Fever (in some cases)

CAUSE
Bacteria enter through cuts, wounds or cracks in skin.

GENERAL PREVENTION TIPS

- Wash hands regularly
- Keep skin clean and dry
- Wear clean, loose clothes
- Avoid sharing personal items
- Keep cuts and wounds clean and covered
- Boost immunity with healthy lifestyle

WHEN TO SEE A DOCTOR?

- Symptoms worsen or don't improve
- Spreading redness or severe pain
- Fever or pus discharge
- Recurring infections

TAKEAWAY

Early care and good hygiene can prevent skin infections and keep your skin healthy.

Myth vs Fact

Myth: All rashes are allergies.
Fact: Many are infections.

Myth: If redness reduces, infection is cured.
Fact: Symptoms may improve without elimination of infection.

Myth: Fungal infections are rare.
Fact: They are very common.

Myth: Warts always need aggressive treatment.
Fact: Some resolve naturally.

Red Flag Warnings

Seek medical advice if you notice:

- Rapidly spreading redness
- Severe pain
- Fever with skin infection
- Blistering rash near the eye
- Persistent or worsening infection
- Recurrent infections

Example: The Wrong Treatment

A 50-year-old man develops an itchy rash on his thigh. He uses a cream meant for eczema.

The redness improves slightly, but the rash spreads.

Evaluation shows a fungal infection.

With proper treatment, the rash resolves.

This example highlights the importance of correct diagnosis.

Key Points

Skin infections are common.

Bacterial infections cause pain, warmth, and swelling.

Fungal infections thrive in moist areas.

Viral infections present in distinct patterns.

Correct diagnosis is essential.

Chapter Summary

Skin infections occur when bacteria, fungi, or viruses affect the skin. They are common and often treatable, but they are frequently misdiagnosed.

Recognizing patterns, understanding symptoms, and using appropriate treatment lead to better outcomes.

Early attention prevents complications and spread.

Action Plan

• Keep skin clean and dry.

• Avoid sharing personal items.

• Treat infections early.

• Do not use random creams.

• Watch for signs of spreading infection.

• Seek medical advice when needed.

• Complete the full course of treatment.

Bridge to the Next Chapter

Infections are important, but many people are more concerned about pigmentation, aging, and long-term skin changes. In the next chapter, we will explore how these changes occur and how to manage and prevent them effectively.

CHAPTER 15: Pigmentation, Aging, and Skin Cancer Prevention — Protecting Your Skin for the Long Term

Changes You Notice, Questions You Ask

At some point, most people begin to notice gradual changes in their skin.

A dark spot that was not there before.
Uneven tone on the face.
Fine lines around the eyes.
Skin that feels thinner or less firm.

These changes raise natural questions.

Is this normal aging?
Is it due to sun exposure?
Can it be reversed?
Should I be concerned?

Some changes are harmless and cosmetic. Others deserve careful attention.

Understanding what is happening helps you respond calmly and correctly.

What Causes Pigmentation

Skin color is determined by melanin, a pigment produced by specialized cells.

When melanin production becomes uneven, pigmentation appears.

Common causes include:

Sun exposure
Inflammation such as acne or rash
Hormonal changes
Aging

Pigmentation may appear as small spots, larger patches, or uneven tone.

Most cases are harmless, but they may take time to improve.

Melasma and Post-Inflammatory Pigmentation

Melasma appears as brown or grayish patches, often on the cheeks, forehead, or upper lip.

It is influenced by hormones and sunlight.

It is more common in women and often appears during periods of hormonal change.

Post-inflammatory pigmentation occurs after acne, injury, or irritation.

It is more noticeable in darker skin tones and may persist for months.

Both conditions require patience and consistent care.

Doctor's Pearl

Without daily sun protection, treatment of pigmentation is incomplete.

Aging Skin: What Truly Changes

Aging is a natural process that affects every layer of the skin.

Collagen gradually decreases, leading to fine lines and wrinkles.

Elastin weakens, reducing the skin's ability to return to its original shape.

Oil production decreases, leading to dryness.

Skin becomes thinner and heals more slowly.

These changes cannot be stopped completely, but they can be slowed.

Photoaging: The Impact of Sun Exposure

Sun exposure is one of the main causes of premature aging.

Over time, repeated exposure leads to:

Wrinkles
Pigmentation
Rough texture
Loss of elasticity
Visible blood vessels

This process is called photoaging.

It develops gradually over years, often without immediate symptoms.

Skin Cancer: Awareness Saves Lives

Skin cancer is a serious condition, but it is often preventable and treatable when detected early.

It may appear as a new growth or a change in an existing lesion.

Awareness is essential.

Early detection significantly improves outcomes.

Recognizing Warning Signs

A useful way to remember suspicious features is to observe:

Asymmetry
Irregular borders
Multiple colors
Increase in size
Change over time

Any lesion that changes should be evaluated.

Other Concerning Features

A sore that does not heal
Bleeding or crusting lesions
Rapidly growing growths
Persistent irritation

These signs require attention.

Doctor's Pearl

A changing skin lesion should never be ignored.

Sun Protection: The Most Effective Prevention

Among all preventive measures, sun protection is the most important.

Use sunscreen regularly.

Protect exposed areas such as the face, neck, and hands.

Wear protective clothing and hats when needed.

Avoid excessive sun exposure, especially during peak hours.

This habit alone can significantly reduce long-term damage.

Treatment of Pigmentation and Aging

Treatment depends on the cause.

Topical treatments may improve pigmentation and texture.

Procedures such as chemical peels or laser therapy may be helpful in selected cases.

Results are gradual.

No treatment provides instant or complete reversal.

Realistic expectations are important.

Common Mistakes to Avoid

Ignoring sun protection
Using multiple strong treatments at once
Expecting rapid results
Using unproven products
Ignoring suspicious skin changes

Myth vs Fact

Myth: Dark spots disappear quickly.
Fact: They often take time.

Myth: Sunscreen is needed only in summer.
Fact: Daily exposure matters year-round.

Myth: Skin cancer occurs only in fair skin.
Fact: It can occur in all skin types.

Myth: Aging can be reversed completely.
Fact: It can be slowed, not reversed.

Red Flag Warnings

Seek medical advice if you notice:

- A changing mole
- A non-healing sore
- Bleeding or crusting lesions
- Rapidly growing growths
- Sudden unusual pigmentation

PIGMENTATION & AGING

UNDERSTAND THE CAUSES. CARE THE RIGHT WAY.

PIGMENTATION

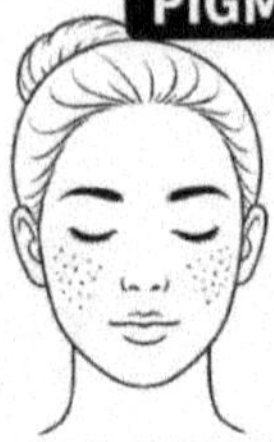

Pigmentation refers to dark spots or uneven skin tone caused by excess melanin production.

TYPES

- Sun spots
- Melasma
- Post-inflammatory hyperpigmentation (PIH)
- Freckles

COMMON CAUSES

- Sun exposure
- Hormonal changes
- Acne or skin injury
- Aging
- Genetics

CARE & MANAGEMENT

- Use broad-spectrum sunscreen daily (SPF 30+)
- Use brightening ingredients (Vitamin C, Niacinamide, Alpha Arbutin, Kojic Acid, Tranexamic Acid)
- Exfoliate gently (AHAs like glycolic acid)
- Be consistent and patient

AGING

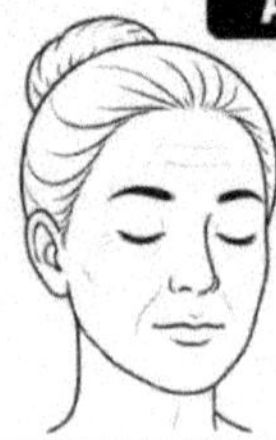

Aging is a natural process that leads to changes in skin texture, elasticity, and appearance.

SIGNS

- Fine lines and wrinkles
- Loss of firmness and elasticity
- Dullness and uneven texture
- Age spots
- Sagging

COMMON CAUSES

- Sun exposure (UV rays)
- Loss of collagen and elastin
- Pollution
- Smoking
- Poor lifestyle (stress, lack of sleep, unhealthy diet)

CARE & MANAGEMENT

- Daily sunscreen (SPF 30+)
- Use anti-aging ingredients (Retinol, Peptides, Vitamin C, Hyaluronic Acid)
- Moisturize and stay hydrated
- Eat a balanced diet and get enough sleep

KEY INGREDIENTS THAT HELP

VITAMIN C
Brightens skin and reduces dark spots

NIACINAMIDE
Fades pigmentation and improves skin tone

RETINOL
Boosts collagen, reduces wrinkles and fine lines

HYALURONIC ACID
Hydrates and plumps the skin

SUNSCREEN
Protects from UV rays and prevents further damage

WHEN TO SEE A DERMATOLOGIST?

- Sudden or excessive darkening of skin
- Pigmentation not improving with home care
- Premature or worsening signs of aging
- Skin irritation or reaction to products

TAKEAWAY

Healthy, even-toned and youthful skin is possible with protection, the right care and consistency.

PROTECT TODAY. CARE DAILY. GLOW FOR LIFE.

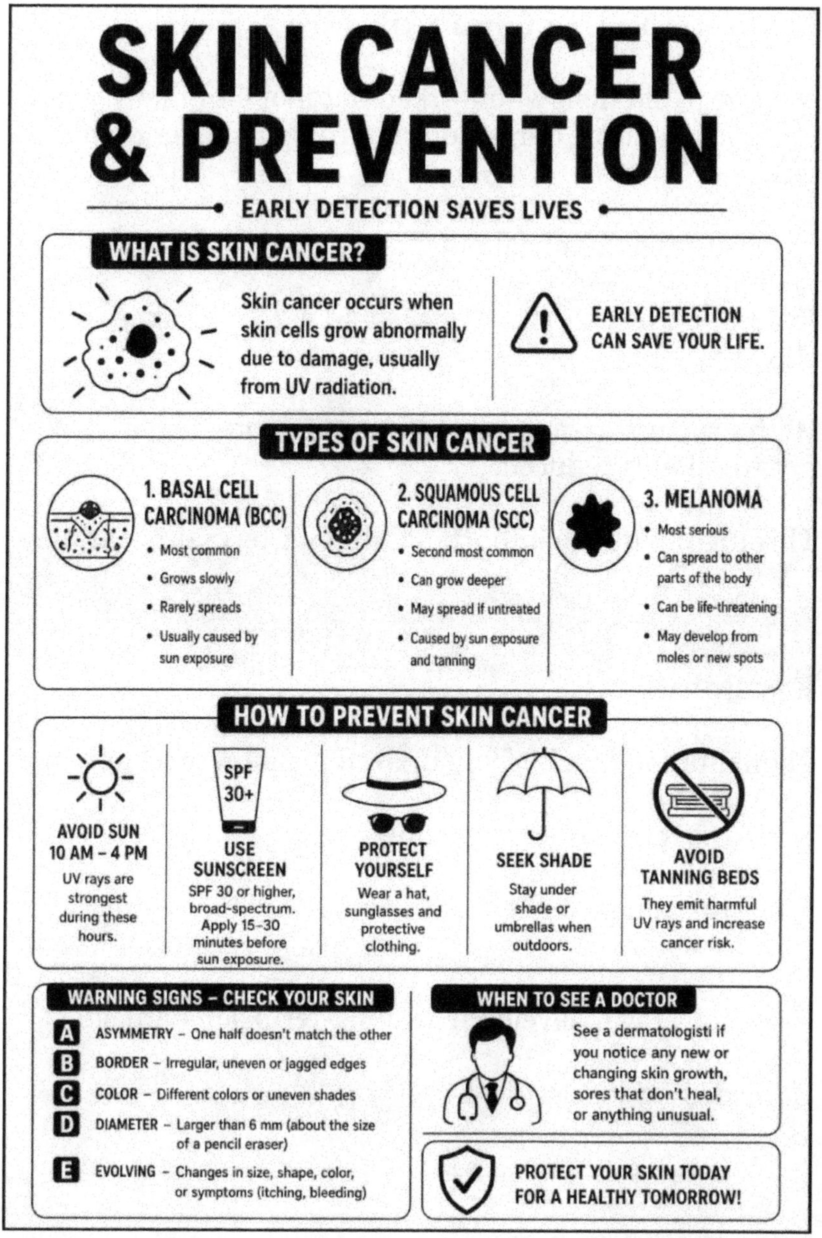
SKIN CANCER
& PREVENTION
EARLY DETECTION SAVES LIVES
WHAT IS SKIN CANCER?
Skin cancer occurs when skin cells grow abnormally due to damage, usually from UV radiation.
EARLY DETECTION CAN SAVE YOUR LIFE.
TYPES OF SKIN CANCER
1. BASAL CELL CARCINOMA (BCC)
• Most common
• Grows slowly
• Rarely spreads
• Usually caused by sun exposure
2. SQUAMOUS CELL CARCINOMA (SCC)
• Second most common
• Can grow deeper
• May spread if untreated
• Caused by sun exposure and tanning
3. MELANOMA
• Most serious
• Can spread to other parts of the body
• Can be life-threatening
• May develop from moles or new spots
HOW TO PREVENT SKIN CANCER
AVOID SUN 10 AM – 4 PM
UV rays are strongest during these hours.
SPF 30+
USE SUNSCREEN
SPF 30 or higher, broad-spectrum. Apply 15–30 minutes before sun exposure.
PROTECT YOURSELF
Wear a hat, sunglasses and protective clothing.
SEEK SHADE
Stay under shade or umbrellas when outdoors.
AVOID TANNING BEDS
They emit harmful UV rays and increase cancer risk.
WARNING SIGNS – CHECK YOUR SKIN
A ASYMMETRY – One half doesn't match the other
B BORDER – Irregular, uneven or jagged edges
C COLOR – Different colors or uneven shades
D DIAMETER – Larger than 6 mm (about the size of a pencil eraser)
E EVOLVING – Changes in size, shape, color, or symptoms (itching, bleeding)
WHEN TO SEE A DOCTOR
See a dermatologisti if you notice any new or changing skin growth, sores that don't heal, or anything unusual.
PROTECT YOUR SKIN TODAY FOR A HEALTHY TOMORROW!

Example: Years of Sun Exposure

A 63-year-old man who worked outdoors for many years develops multiple dark spots and rough patches on his face.

Some areas do not heal.

Evaluation reveals sun damage and early precancerous changes.

With proper treatment and sun protection, further progression is reduced.

This highlights the importance of long-term prevention.

Key Points

Pigmentation results from uneven melanin production.

Sun exposure accelerates aging.

Melasma and post-inflammatory pigmentation are common.

Skin cancer can develop from long-term sun damage.

Early detection is critical.

Chapter Summary

Pigmentation and aging are natural processes influenced by sun exposure, hormones, and time. While many changes are harmless, some may indicate serious conditions.

Sun protection, early recognition of warning signs, and appropriate treatment are essential.

Understanding these changes allows for better prevention and long-term care.

Action Plan

- Use sunscreen daily.
- Protect your skin from excessive sun exposure.
- Observe changes in moles and lesions.
- Use appropriate treatments with patience.
- Avoid overuse of strong products.
- Seek medical advice for suspicious changes.
- Focus on long-term prevention.

Bridge to the Next Chapter

While skin concerns are common, hair loss remains one of the most distressing problems for many people. In the next chapter, we will explore different types of hair loss, their causes, and what truly works.

CHAPTER 16: Hair Loss — Causes, Patterns, and What Truly Works

A Concern That Feels Personal

Hair loss is one of the most common concerns I hear in the clinic.

It often begins quietly. A few extra strands on the pillow. More hair in the shower drain. A slightly wider part. A receding hairline that is easy to ignore at first.

Then, gradually, it becomes difficult to ignore.

Hair is not just about appearance. It is closely tied to identity and confidence. That is why even mild changes can feel significant.

The important thing to remember is this.

Hair loss is not one condition. It has many causes. Understanding the type is the key to managing it correctly.

Understanding the Pattern

Hair loss rarely occurs without a pattern.

Gradual thinning over time suggests one cause.

Sudden increased shedding suggests another.

Patchy hair loss suggests something different.

Careful observation helps guide the diagnosis.

Pattern Hair Loss: The Most Common Type

This is the most common form of hair loss.

In men, it usually begins with a receding hairline and thinning at the crown.

In women, it appears as gradual thinning over the top of the scalp, with widening of the part.

This type is influenced by genetics and hormones.

It develops slowly over time.

Early treatment can slow progression.

Doctor's Pearl

Hair loss that is recognized early is easier to manage.

Telogen Effluvium: Sudden Shedding

This condition causes noticeable increase in hair shedding.

It usually occurs two to three months after a triggering event such as:

Severe illness
Surgery
Emotional stress
Rapid weight loss
Childbirth

Hair follicles shift into the shedding phase.

The shedding can be alarming, but it is usually temporary.

As the body recovers, hair growth gradually returns.

Alopecia Areata: Patchy Loss

This is an autoimmune condition.

It causes sudden, well-defined patches of hair loss.

The skin in these areas appears smooth.

The course is unpredictable. Hair may regrow, or new patches may appear.

Early evaluation is important.

Nutritional and Hormonal Causes

Hair growth depends on overall health.

Iron deficiency is a common cause of hair thinning.

Thyroid disorders can affect hair growth and texture.

Hormonal imbalance, especially in women, may cause scalp hair thinning and increased facial hair.

Correcting the underlying cause improves outcomes.

Scarring Hair Loss: When Follicles Are Damaged

Some forms of hair loss involve damage to the hair follicle.

These are called scarring alopecias.

They may present with redness, pain, or scaling.

If untreated, hair loss may become permanent.

Early diagnosis is critical.

Hair Care Practices That Affect Hair Health

Daily habits matter.

Tight hairstyles can pull on hair follicles and lead to traction hair loss.

Frequent use of heat tools weakens the hair shaft.

Chemical treatments can damage hair over time.

Gentle handling helps preserve hair strength.

Treatment Options: What Helps

Treatment depends on the cause.

Topical treatments may help stimulate hair growth.

Oral medications may be useful in selected cases.

Treating underlying medical conditions is important.

In some cases, procedures such as hair transplant may be considered.

No single treatment works for all types.

Hair Oils and Supplements: Setting Realistic Expectations

Hair oils improve dryness and shine.

They do not treat most types of hair loss.

Supplements help only if there is a deficiency.

Relying only on oils or supplements often leads to disappointment.

Patience and Consistency

Hair grows slowly.

Visible improvement takes time.

Many treatments require several months before results are noticeable.

Stopping treatment too early is a common mistake.

Common Mistakes to Avoid

Ignoring early signs
Switching treatments frequently
Expecting quick results
Using multiple treatments without guidance
Relying only on home remedies

Myth vs Fact

Myth: Hair loss is always permanent.
Fact: Many types are temporary or manageable.

Myth: Oils can regrow hair.
Fact: They improve hair texture, not most causes.

Myth: Washing hair causes hair loss.
Fact: It removes hair that is already shedding.

Myth: Supplements always help.
Fact: Only when deficiency exists.

Red Flag Warnings

Seek medical advice if you notice:

- Sudden heavy shedding
- Patchy hair loss
- Hair loss with scalp pain or redness
- Hair loss with fatigue or weight change
- Loss of eyebrows or body hair

Example: Early vs Late Action

A 42-year-old man notices gradual thinning at the crown but ignores it.

Several years later, hair loss has progressed significantly.

When treatment is started earlier, the outcome is usually better.

This highlights the importance of timely attention.

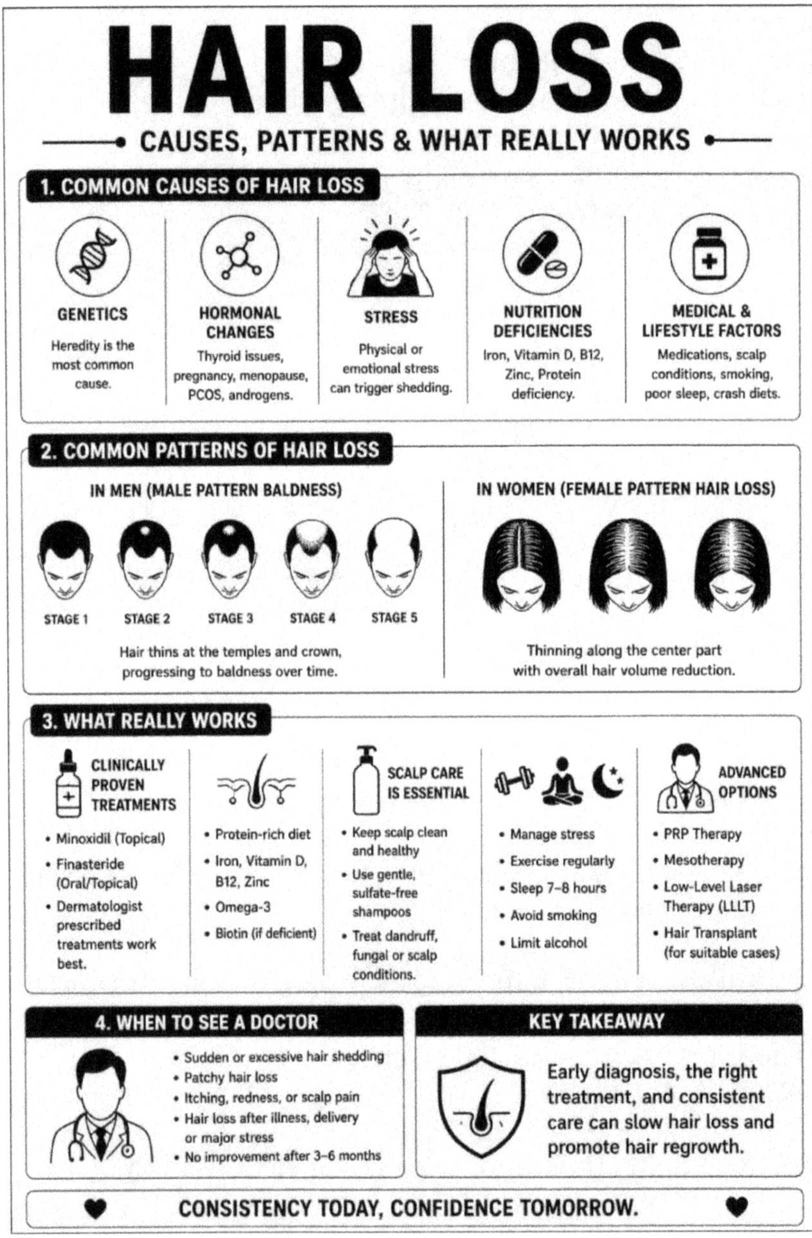
HAIR LOSS
CAUSES, PATTERNS & WHAT REALLY WORKS
1. COMMON CAUSES OF HAIR LOSS
GENETICS
Heredity is the most common cause.
HORMONAL CHANGES
Thyroid issues, pregnancy, menopause, PCOS, androgens.
STRESS
Physical or emotional stress can trigger shedding.
NUTRITION DEFICIENCIES
Iron, Vitamin D, B12, Zinc, Protein deficiency.
MEDICAL & LIFESTYLE FACTORS
Medications, scalp conditions, smoking, poor sleep, crash diets.
2. COMMON PATTERNS OF HAIR LOSS
IN MEN (MALE PATTERN BALDNESS)
STAGE 1
STAGE 2
STAGE 3
STAGE 4
STAGE 5
Hair thins at the temples and crown, progressing to baldness over time.
IN WOMEN (FEMALE PATTERN HAIR LOSS)
Thinning along the center part with overall hair volume reduction.
3. WHAT REALLY WORKS
CLINICALLY PROVEN TREATMENTS
• Minoxidil (Topical)
• Finasteride (Oral/Topical)
• Dermatologist prescribed treatments work best.
• Protein-rich diet
• Iron, Vitamin D, B12, Zinc
• Omega-3
• Biotin (if deficient)
SCALP CARE IS ESSENTIAL
• Keep scalp clean and healthy
• Use gentle, sulfate-free shampoos
• Treat dandruff, fungal or scalp conditions.
• Manage stress
• Exercise regularly
• Sleep 7–8 hours
• Avoid smoking
• Limit alcohol
ADVANCED OPTIONS
• PRP Therapy
• Mesotherapy
• Low-Level Laser Therapy (LLLT)
• Hair Transplant (for suitable cases)
4. WHEN TO SEE A DOCTOR
• Sudden or excessive hair shedding
• Patchy hair loss
• Itching, redness, or scalp pain
• Hair loss after illness, delivery or major stress
• No improvement after 3–6 months
KEY TAKEAWAY
Early diagnosis, the right treatment, and consistent care can slow hair loss and promote hair regrowth.
CONSISTENCY TODAY, CONFIDENCE TOMORROW.

Key Points

Hair loss has multiple causes.

Pattern hair loss is common and progressive.

Sudden shedding is often temporary.

Some conditions can become permanent if untreated.

Early diagnosis improves outcomes.

Chapter Summary

Hair loss is a multifactorial condition influenced by genetics, hormones, stress, nutrition, and health. Different patterns indicate different causes.

Some types are temporary, while others require long-term management.

Early evaluation, appropriate treatment, and patience are essential for better results.

Action Plan

- Observe your hair loss pattern.

- Note recent stress, illness, or weight changes.

- Avoid tight hairstyles and excessive heat.

- Use gentle hair care.
- Do not rely only on oils or supplements.
- Seek medical advice for persistent or unusual hair loss.
- Follow treatment consistently.
- Be patient with results.

Bridge to the Next Chapter

Hair health is closely linked to the scalp. In the next chapter, we will focus on scalp conditions such as dandruff, inflammation, and infections, and how they affect hair growth.

CHAPTER 17: Scalp Disorders and Hair Care Mistakes — Fix the Root, Not Just the Hair

Why the Scalp Deserves Your Attention

Many people focus on the hair they see.

Shine, thickness, style, color.

But the real story begins at the scalp.

If the scalp is unhealthy, hair cannot grow well. It may shed more, feel weaker, or look dull no matter how many products are used.

Think of it like soil and a plant. Healthy soil supports growth. Poor soil limits it.

The same is true for your scalp.

Dandruff: Common, Persistent, and Often Misunderstood

Dandruff is one of the most common scalp problems.

It appears as white or yellowish flakes on the scalp and sometimes on the shoulders. It may be associated with itching.

Many people assume dandruff is simply due to dry skin.

In reality, it is often related to a mild inflammatory response to natural yeast that lives on the scalp.

This is why dandruff may come and go and may worsen with stress or weather changes.

Regular use of appropriate shampoos usually controls it.

Doctor's Pearl

Flaking with itching often reflects inflammation, not just dryness.

Seborrheic Dermatitis: A More Active Form

Seborrheic dermatitis is a more persistent and sometimes more noticeable form of dandruff.

It may affect not only the scalp but also:

Eyebrows
Sides of the nose
Behind the ears

The skin may appear red with greasy scales.

It tends to flare with stress, fatigue, or environmental changes.

Treatment is similar to dandruff but may require additional measures.

Scalp Psoriasis: Thick and Well-Defined

Psoriasis can involve the scalp.

It presents as thick, well-defined patches with silvery scales.

It may extend beyond the hairline.

Itching may be present.

It is often confused with dandruff, but it behaves differently and may require specific treatment.

Fungal Infections of the Scalp

Fungal infections can affect the scalp and may lead to:

Scaling
Itching
Patchy hair loss

These infections require proper diagnosis and treatment.

Using incorrect products may worsen the condition or delay recovery.

Folliculitis: Inflammation of Hair Follicles

Folliculitis appears as small red or pus-filled bumps on the scalp.

It may be caused by bacteria, irritation, or friction.

It can cause discomfort and sometimes mild hair loss in affected areas.

Good hygiene and appropriate treatment usually help.

Traction Hair Loss: A Preventable Problem

Certain hairstyles place continuous tension on the hair.

Over time, this can damage the hair follicles.

Common causes include:

Tight ponytails
Braids
Buns
Hair extensions

Early stages are reversible.

Long-term traction can lead to permanent hair loss.

Damage from Heat and Chemicals

Frequent use of heat tools weakens the hair shaft.

Chemical treatments such as coloring, perming, or straightening can damage hair over time.

These do not directly affect the hair root, but they make the hair more prone to breakage.

Moderation is essential.

Product Overuse and Scalp Buildup

Using too many hair products can lead to buildup.

This may cause:

Itching
Flaking
Irritation

Some products may clog follicles or worsen existing scalp conditions.

A simpler routine often works better.

Hair Washing: Finding Balance

Many people are unsure how often to wash their hair.

The answer depends on the scalp.

An oily scalp may require more frequent washing.

A dry or sensitive scalp may need less frequent washing with gentle products.

Both over-washing and under-washing can cause problems.

Doctor's Pearl

Wash based on your scalp condition, not on a fixed schedule.

Common Mistakes to Avoid

Ignoring scalp symptoms
Using harsh shampoos
Keeping tight hairstyles for long periods
Excessive heat styling
Using too many products
Delaying treatment for infections

Myth vs Fact

Myth: Dandruff is caused by dryness alone.
Fact: It is often related to inflammation and yeast.

Myth: Oiling the scalp cures dandruff.
Fact: It may sometimes worsen it.

Myth: Washing hair causes hair loss.
Fact: It removes hair that is already shedding.

Myth: All scalp flaking is the same.
Fact: Different conditions require different treatment.

Red Flag Warnings

Seek medical advice if you notice:

- Severe or persistent itching
- Thick scaling or redness
- Patchy hair loss
- Painful scalp lesions
- Pus-filled bumps
- No improvement with basic care

Example: A Simple Change That Matters

A 40-year-old woman regularly wears tight hairstyles. She notices thinning along the hairline.

This is traction hair loss.

When she changes her styling habits early, further damage is prevented.

This shows how daily habits can affect long-term outcomes.

HAIR CARE MISTAKES

AVOID TODAY. PROTECT YOUR HAIR TOMORROW.

COMMON HAIR CARE MISTAKES

1 OVERWASHING YOUR HAIR
Washes away natural oils, causing dryness, frizz and scalp irritation.

2 USING HOT WATER
Strips moisture and weakens hair, leading to dullness and breakage.

3 HARSH CHEMICALS
Sulfates, parabens and strong chemicals can damage hair and scalp.

4 OVER-STYLING WITH HEAT
Frequent use of heat tools causes heat damage, split ends and breakage.

5 TIGHT HAIRSTYLES
Pulls on hair roots and can lead to hair fall and breakage.

6 IGNORING SCALP HEALTH
A dirty or unhealthy scalp can cause dandruff, itching and hair loss.

7 SKIPPING CONDITIONER
Makes hair dry, rough and more prone to tangles and breakage.

8 WRONG PRODUCTS
Using products not suited for your hair type can cause buildup and damage.

9 TOO MUCH PRODUCT
Overuse of gels, serums or sprays weighs hair down and causes buildup.

10 POOR DIET & HYDRATION
Lack of nutrients and water weakens hair and slows growth.

WHAT TO DO INSTEAD

- Wash 2–3 times a week.
- Use lukewarm or cool water.
- Choose mild, sulfate-free products.
- Limit heat styling. Use heat protectant when needed.
- Use gentle hairstyles.
- Keep scalp clean and well-nourished.
- Eat a balanced diet and drink plenty of water.

HEALTHY HAIR HABITS

- Oil your hair regularly
- Trim your hair every 6–8 weeks
- Detangle gently, starting from the ends
- Use a soft microfiber towel
- Get enough sleep and manage stress
- Be consistent and patient

REMEMBER

Good hair care is not about using more products, it's about using the right care and being consistent.

TAKE CARE OF YOUR HAIR TODAY FOR A HEALTHIER, STRONGER TOMORROW!

Key Points

Scalp health is essential for healthy hair.

Dandruff and seborrheic dermatitis are common.

Scalp psoriasis and infections require proper diagnosis.

Tight hairstyles can cause hair loss.

Simple habits make a significant difference.

Chapter Summary

The scalp plays a central role in hair health. Conditions such as dandruff, seborrheic dermatitis, psoriasis, infections, and folliculitis can affect the scalp and hair growth.

Daily habits such as tight hairstyles, excessive heat, and product overuse can damage hair and scalp.

Understanding and addressing these factors helps maintain healthier hair.

Action Plan

- Pay attention to scalp health.

- Use appropriate shampoos.

- Avoid tight hairstyles.
- Limit heat and chemical treatments.
- Keep your routine simple.
- Treat scalp problems early.
- Seek medical advice when needed.

Bridge to the Next Chapter

Skin and hair concerns often differ between individuals. In the next chapter, we will focus on skin and hair health in women, including hormonal influences and changes across different life stages.

CHAPTER 18: Skin and Hair Health in Women — Understanding Hormones, Life Stages, and Real Solutions

Changes That Follow a Pattern

Women often notice that their skin and hair do not remain the same throughout life.

There are phases when the skin feels clear and balanced. Then there are times when acne appears, hair sheds more, or pigmentation becomes noticeable.

These changes are not random.

They often follow hormonal patterns linked to different life stages such as puberty, menstrual cycles, pregnancy, postpartum period, and menopause.

When you understand these patterns, you begin to feel more in control.

Hormones and Their Visible Effects

Hormones influence many aspects of skin and hair.

They affect oil production, pigmentation, hair growth, and hair shedding.

Even small changes in hormone levels can lead to noticeable effects.

This is why some problems appear suddenly and then improve, only to return again.

Adult Acne: Not Just a Teenage Problem

Many women develop acne in adulthood.

It often appears along the jawline, chin, and neck.

It may worsen before menstrual cycles.

This type of acne is often driven by hormonal changes.

It tends to be persistent and may require a different approach than teenage acne.

Gentle care and appropriate treatment are important.

Doctor's Pearl

Adult acne often needs patience and a targeted approach, not aggressive treatment.

Melasma and Pigmentation

Melasma is a common concern.

It appears as brown or grayish patches on the face, especially on the cheeks, forehead, and upper lip.

It is influenced by hormones and sun exposure.

It may develop during pregnancy or with hormonal fluctuations.

Post-inflammatory pigmentation after acne or irritation is also common.

Both conditions take time to improve and require consistent sun protection.

Pregnancy and Skin Changes

Pregnancy brings visible changes.

Some women notice a natural glow due to increased blood flow.

Others may develop acne, pigmentation, or sensitivity.

Stretch marks may appear as the skin expands.

Hair may appear thicker during pregnancy because fewer hairs enter the shedding phase.

Most of these changes are temporary.

Postpartum Hair Loss: A Temporary Phase

After delivery, many women experience increased hair shedding.

This usually begins two to three months after childbirth.

Hair that remained in the growth phase during pregnancy shifts into the shedding phase.

This can be distressing, but it is usually temporary.

Hair growth gradually returns to normal.

Polycystic Ovarian Syndrome (PCOS)

PCOS is a common hormonal condition.

It may present with:

Persistent acne
Excess facial hair
Hair thinning on the scalp
Irregular menstrual cycles

These changes are related to hormonal imbalance.

Management often includes lifestyle changes and medical treatment.

Menopause and Skin Aging

Menopause brings a gradual decline in hormone levels.

Skin becomes thinner, drier, and less elastic.

Wrinkles may become more noticeable.

Hair may become thinner.

These changes are natural.

Proper skin care, nutrition, and lifestyle habits help manage them.

Hair Thinning in Women

Hair thinning in women usually presents as a reduction in density.

The part becomes wider, but the front hairline is often preserved.

This type of hair loss is influenced by genetics and hormones.

Early treatment can help slow progression.

Unwanted Hair Growth

Some women notice increased hair growth on the face or body.

This may be due to hormonal changes.

Evaluation is important to identify the cause.

Treatment depends on the underlying condition.

The Emotional Impact

Skin and hair changes can affect confidence.

Many women feel uncomfortable discussing these concerns.

It is important to recognize that these concerns are valid.

Addressing them improves both physical and emotional well-being.

Common Mistakes to Avoid

Ignoring hormonal patterns
Using multiple products without guidance
Expecting quick results
Delaying medical evaluation
Relying only on home remedies

Myth vs Fact

Myth: Adult acne is rare.
Fact: It is very common.

Myth: Hair loss after pregnancy is permanent.
Fact: It is usually temporary.

Myth: Pigmentation can be removed quickly.
Fact: It often takes time.

Myth: Hormonal problems always require complex treatment.
Fact: Many are manageable.

Red Flag Warnings

Seek medical advice if you notice:

- Severe or persistent acne
- Sudden hair thinning
- Excess facial hair with other symptoms
- Irregular menstrual cycles with skin changes
- Rapid pigmentation changes

Example: Understanding Postpartum Changes

A 33-year-old woman notices heavy hair shedding a few months after childbirth.

She fears permanent hair loss.

Once she understands the normal postpartum pattern, her anxiety reduces.

With time, her hair growth returns to normal.

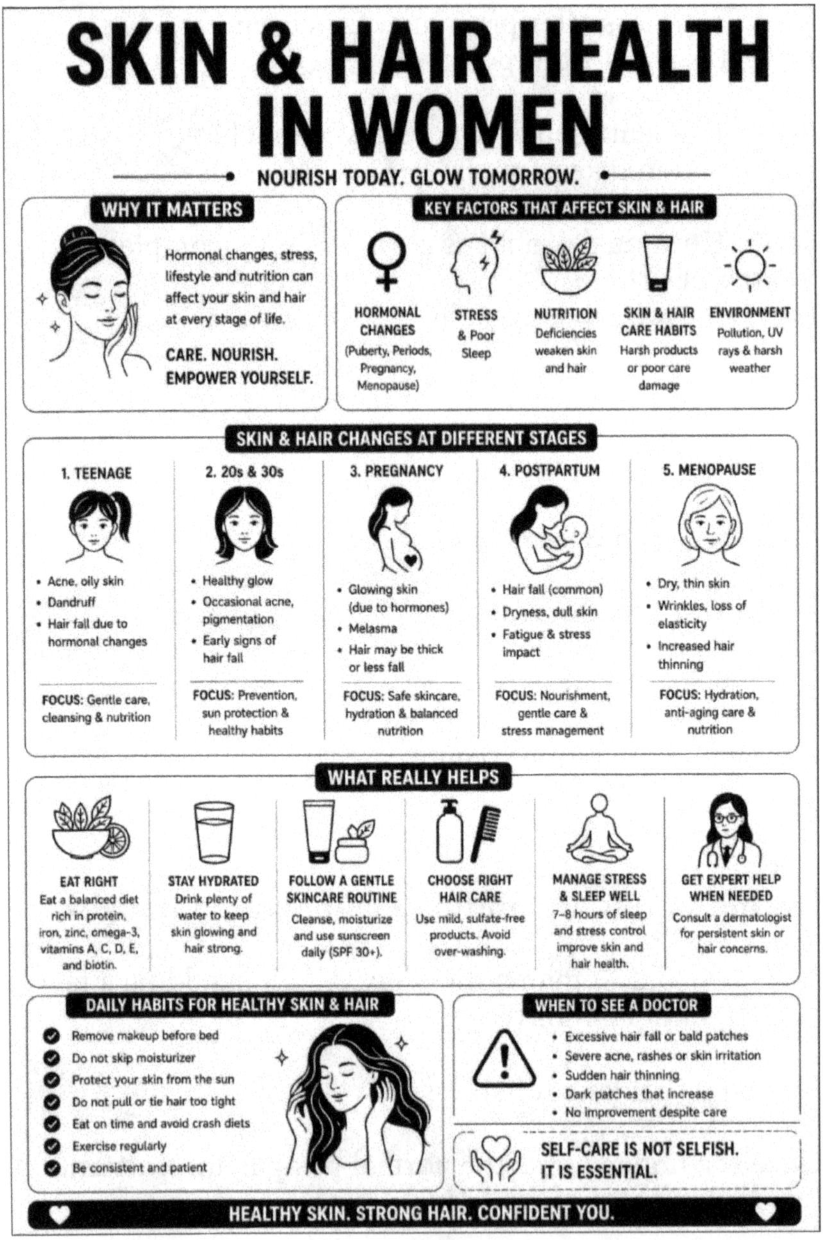
SKIN & HAIR HEALTH IN WOMEN
NOURISH TODAY. GLOW TOMORROW.
WHY IT MATTERS
Hormonal changes, stress, lifestyle and nutrition can affect your skin and hair at every stage of life.
CARE. NOURISH. EMPOWER YOURSELF.
KEY FACTORS THAT AFFECT SKIN & HAIR
HORMONAL CHANGES (Puberty, Periods, Pregnancy, Menopause)
STRESS & Poor Sleep
NUTRITION Deficiencies weaken skin and hair
SKIN & HAIR CARE HABITS Harsh products or poor care damage
ENVIRONMENT Pollution, UV rays & harsh weather
SKIN & HAIR CHANGES AT DIFFERENT STAGES
1. TEENAGE
• Acne, oily skin
• Dandruff
• Hair fall due to hormonal changes
FOCUS: Gentle care, cleansing & nutrition
2. 20s & 30s
• Healthy glow
• Occasional acne, pigmentation
• Early signs of hair fall
FOCUS: Prevention, sun protection & healthy habits
3. PREGNANCY
• Glowing skin (due to hormones)
• Melasma
• Hair may be thick or less fall
FOCUS: Safe skincare, hydration & balanced nutrition
4. POSTPARTUM
• Hair fall (common)
• Dryness, dull skin
• Fatigue & stress impact
FOCUS: Nourishment, gentle care & stress management
5. MENOPAUSE
• Dry, thin skin
• Wrinkles, loss of elasticity
• Increased hair thinning
FOCUS: Hydration, anti-aging care & nutrition
WHAT REALLY HELPS
EAT RIGHT Eat a balanced diet rich in protein, iron, zinc, omega-3, vitamins A, C, D, E, and biotin.
STAY HYDRATED Drink plenty of water to keep skin glowing and hair strong.
FOLLOW A GENTLE SKINCARE ROUTINE Cleanse, moisturize and use sunscreen daily (SPF 30+).
CHOOSE RIGHT HAIR CARE Use mild, sulfate-free products. Avoid over-washing.
MANAGE STRESS & SLEEP WELL 7–8 hours of sleep and stress control improve skin and hair health.
GET EXPERT HELP WHEN NEEDED Consult a dermatologist for persistent skin or hair concerns.
DAILY HABITS FOR HEALTHY SKIN & HAIR
Remove makeup before bed
Do not skip moisturizer
Protect your skin from the sun
Do not pull or tie hair too tight
Eat on time and avoid crash diets
Exercise regularly
Be consistent and patient
WHEN TO SEE A DOCTOR
• Excessive hair fall or bald patches
• Severe acne, rashes or skin irritation
• Sudden hair thinning
• Dark patches that increase
• No improvement despite care
SELF-CARE IS NOT SELFISH. IT IS ESSENTIAL.
HEALTHY SKIN. STRONG HAIR. CONFIDENT YOU.

Key Points

Hormones play a major role in women's skin and hair.

Life stages bring predictable changes.

Many changes are temporary or manageable.

Early recognition helps guide care.

Chapter Summary

Skin and hair health in women is influenced by hormonal changes across different life stages. Acne, pigmentation, hair thinning, and unwanted hair growth are common concerns.

Pregnancy, postpartum changes, PCOS, and menopause each bring specific patterns.

Understanding these patterns allows for better management and more realistic expectations.

Action Plan

- Observe patterns related to hormonal changes.

- Use gentle and consistent skin care.

- Protect your skin from sun exposure.

- Maintain balanced nutrition.
- Seek medical advice for persistent symptoms.
- Be patient with life-stage changes.
- Focus on long-term care.

Bridge to the Next Chapter

Men also have specific skin and hair concerns, though they are often handled differently. In the next chapter, we will focus on skin and hair health in men and practical ways to manage common problems.

CHAPTER 19: Skin and Hair Health in Men — Practical Care That Works

A Simple Approach, Often Overlooked

Many men prefer to keep things simple.

That is not a problem. In fact, it is often an advantage.

The difficulty is not simplicity. The difficulty is neglect.

Small issues are ignored. Early signs are dismissed. Quick fixes are tried without understanding the cause.

Over time, these habits allow problems such as hair loss, shaving irritation, acne, and sun damage to become more noticeable.

The goal of this chapter is not to complicate your routine. It is to make it effective.

Male Pattern Hair Loss: Recognize It Early

Hair loss is the most common concern in men.

It usually follows a clear pattern:

A receding hairline
Thinning at the crown
Gradual progression over time

This is influenced by genetics and hormones.

Many men assume nothing can be done. That is not entirely true.

Early attention can slow progression and improve appearance.

Doctor's Pearl

Hair loss managed early gives better results than hair loss ignored.

Shaving Problems: Small Changes, Big Difference

Shaving is a daily routine for many men.

Improper technique can lead to:

Razor burns
Irritation
Ingrown hairs
Small bumps

These problems often occur due to:

Using dull blades
Shaving too closely
Shaving against the direction of hair growth
Lack of lubrication

Simple changes can reduce these problems significantly.

Beard and Underlying Skin Care

A beard does not eliminate the need for skin care.

The skin under the beard can become dry, irritated, or flaky.

Regular cleansing and occasional conditioning help maintain both skin and hair.

Keeping the beard clean and trimmed reduces discomfort.

Acne in Men

Acne may persist into adulthood.

Shaving can worsen acne by irritating the skin.

Using gentle products and proper shaving technique helps.

Moderate or severe acne requires appropriate treatment.

Sun Exposure: A Commonly Ignored Risk

Many men spend time outdoors for work or activity.

Sun exposure over time leads to:

Pigmentation
Wrinkles
Rough texture
Increased risk of skin cancer

Men are less likely to use sunscreen regularly.

This increases long-term risk.

Daily sun protection is important.

Scalp Care

Scalp problems such as dandruff and itching are common.

Ignoring them leads to discomfort and may affect hair quality.

Regular washing with appropriate shampoo helps maintain scalp health.

Sweat, Friction, and Skin Problems

Sweating is natural.

However, when combined with friction and moisture, it can lead to:

Rashes
Infections
Irritation

Keeping the skin clean and dry helps prevent these issues.

Lifestyle Habits That Matter

Certain habits gradually affect skin and hair.

Smoking accelerates aging and reduces blood flow.

Alcohol affects hydration.

Poor diet weakens overall health.

Irregular sleep and stress increase inflammation.

Improving these habits has long-term benefits.

Common Mistakes to Avoid

Ignoring early hair loss
Using harsh soaps
Poor shaving technique
Skipping sunscreen
Ignoring scalp problems
Neglecting lifestyle habits

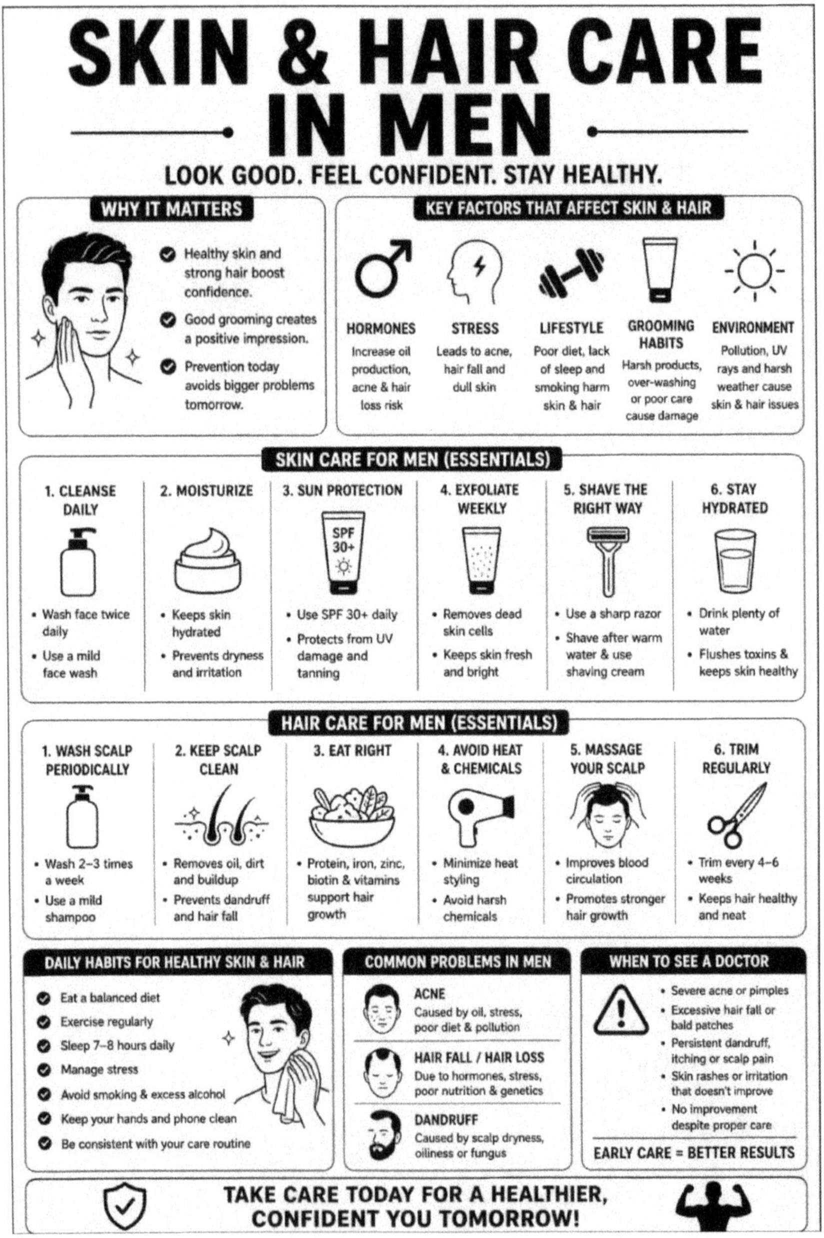
SKIN & HAIR CARE
IN MEN
LOOK GOOD. FEEL CONFIDENT. STAY HEALTHY.
WHY IT MATTERS
Healthy skin and strong hair boost confidence.
Good grooming creates a positive impression.
Prevention today avoids bigger problems tomorrow.
KEY FACTORS THAT AFFECT SKIN & HAIR
HORMONES
Increase oil production, acne & hair loss risk
STRESS
Leads to acne, hair fall and dull skin
LIFESTYLE
Poor diet, lack of sleep and smoking harm skin & hair
GROOMING HABITS
Harsh products, over-washing or poor care cause damage
ENVIRONMENT
Pollution, UV rays and harsh weather cause skin & hair issues
SKIN CARE FOR MEN (ESSENTIALS)
1. CLEANSE DAILY
• Wash face twice daily
• Use a mild face wash
2. MOISTURIZE
• Keeps skin hydrated
• Prevents dryness and irritation
3. SUN PROTECTION
SPF 30+
• Use SPF 30+ daily
• Protects from UV damage and tanning
4. EXFOLIATE WEEKLY
• Removes dead skin cells
• Keeps skin fresh and bright
5. SHAVE THE RIGHT WAY
• Use a sharp razor
• Shave after warm water & use shaving cream
6. STAY HYDRATED
• Drink plenty of water
• Flushes toxins & keeps skin healthy
HAIR CARE FOR MEN (ESSENTIALS)
1. WASH SCALP PERIODICALLY
• Wash 2–3 times a week
• Use a mild shampoo
2. KEEP SCALP CLEAN
• Removes oil, dirt and buildup
• Prevents dandruff and hair fall
3. EAT RIGHT
• Protein, iron, zinc, biotin & vitamins support hair growth
4. AVOID HEAT & CHEMICALS
• Minimize heat styling
• Avoid harsh chemicals
5. MASSAGE YOUR SCALP
• Improves blood circulation
• Promotes stronger hair growth
6. TRIM REGULARLY
• Trim every 4–6 weeks
• Keeps hair healthy and neat
DAILY HABITS FOR HEALTHY SKIN & HAIR
Eat a balanced diet
Exercise regularly
Sleep 7–8 hours daily
Manage stress
Avoid smoking & excess alcohol
Keep your hands and phone clean
Be consistent with your care routine
COMMON PROBLEMS IN MEN
ACNE
Caused by oil, stress, poor diet & pollution
HAIR FALL / HAIR LOSS
Due to hormones, stress, poor nutrition & genetics
DANDRUFF
Caused by scalp dryness, oiliness or fungus
WHEN TO SEE A DOCTOR
• Severe acne or pimples
• Excessive hair fall or bald patches
• Persistent dandruff, itching or scalp pain
• Skin rashes or irritation that doesn't improve
• No improvement despite proper care
EARLY CARE = BETTER RESULTS
TAKE CARE TODAY FOR A HEALTHIER, CONFIDENT YOU TOMORROW!

Myth vs Fact

Myth: Hair loss in men cannot be managed.
Fact: Early treatment can slow progression.

Myth: Men do not need skin care.
Fact: Basic care is important.

Myth: Shaving makes hair grow thicker.
Fact: Hair thickness is determined by the follicle.

Myth: Sunscreen is unnecessary for men.
Fact: It is essential for all.

Red Flag Warnings

Seek medical advice if you notice:

- Rapid hair loss
- Painful or inflamed scalp
- Persistent acne
- Non-healing skin lesions
- Changing moles

Example: A Missed Opportunity

A 41-year-old man notices thinning hair but ignores it.

Several years later, hair loss becomes more advanced.

Earlier treatment could have slowed progression.

This shows the value of timely attention.

Key Points

Hair loss is common in men.

Shaving technique affects skin health.

Sun protection is often overlooked.

Scalp care is important.

Simple habits make a difference.

Chapter Summary

Men often approach skin and hair care simply, but this simplicity should not become neglect. Common concerns such as hair loss, shaving irritation, acne, sun exposure, and scalp problems can be managed effectively with basic, consistent care.

Early recognition and practical habits lead to better long-term outcomes.

Action Plan

- Observe early signs of hair loss.

- Improve shaving technique.
- Use a simple skin care routine.
- Protect your skin from sun exposure.
- Maintain scalp hygiene.
- Improve lifestyle habits.
- Seek medical advice when needed.

Bridge to the Next Chapter

Now that we understand the specific needs of men and women, the next step is to look at treatment options in a structured way. In the next chapter, we will explore medical, cosmetic, and surgical treatments and how to choose wisely.

CHAPTER 20: Medical, Cosmetic, and Surgical Treatments — Choosing Wisely

Not Every Problem Needs a Strong Treatment

By this stage, you understand your skin and hair better.

You know the causes, the patterns, the warning signs, and the role of lifestyle.

Now comes the next question.

What treatment should I choose?

This is where many people feel overwhelmed.

There are creams, tablets, procedures, devices, and surgeries. Some are highly effective. Some are helpful only in selected situations. Some are unnecessary.

The goal is not to choose the strongest treatment.

The goal is to choose the right treatment.

Start with the Right Diagnosis

Before any treatment begins, one step is essential.

Know what you are treating.

A fungal infection treated as eczema will not improve.

Hair loss due to stress will not respond to the same treatment as pattern hair loss.

Correct diagnosis simplifies treatment.

Doctor's Pearl

The right diagnosis reduces unnecessary treatment.

Topical Treatments: The First Line

Most skin and scalp conditions are treated initially with topical medications.

These include creams, gels, lotions, and solutions applied directly to the skin.

They may work by:

Reducing inflammation
Controlling infection
Improving skin turnover
Repairing the skin barrier

Topical treatments are often effective and relatively safe when used correctly.

However, incorrect use can cause irritation or poor results.

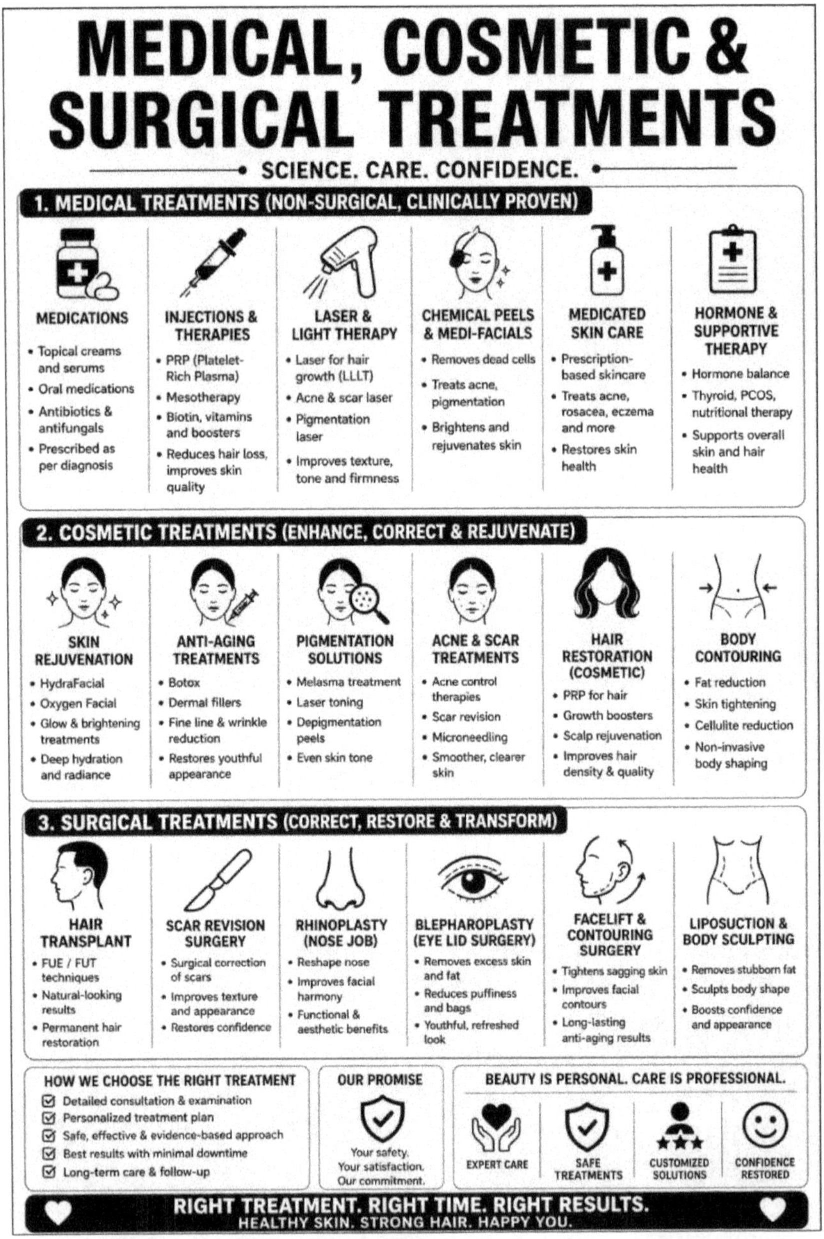
MEDICAL, COSMETIC & SURGICAL TREATMENTS
SCIENCE. CARE. CONFIDENCE.
1. MEDICAL TREATMENTS (NON-SURGICAL, CLINICALLY PROVEN)
MEDICATIONS
• Topical creams and serums
• Oral medications
• Antibiotics & antifungals
• Prescribed as per diagnosis
INJECTIONS & THERAPIES
• PRP (Platelet-Rich Plasma)
• Mesotherapy
• Biotin, vitamins and boosters
• Reduces hair loss, improves skin quality
LASER & LIGHT THERAPY
• Laser for hair growth (LLLT)
• Acne & scar laser
• Pigmentation laser
• Improves texture, tone and firmness
CHEMICAL PEELS & MEDI-FACIALS
• Removes dead cells
• Treats acne, pigmentation
• Brightens and rejuvenates skin
MEDICATED SKIN CARE
• Prescription-based skincare
• Treats acne, rosacea, eczema and more
• Restores skin health
HORMONE & SUPPORTIVE THERAPY
• Hormone balance
• Thyroid, PCOS, nutritional therapy
• Supports overall skin and hair health
2. COSMETIC TREATMENTS (ENHANCE, CORRECT & REJUVENATE)
SKIN REJUVENATION
• HydraFacial
• Oxygen Facial
• Glow & brightening treatments
• Deep hydration and radiance
ANTI-AGING TREATMENTS
• Botox
• Dermal fillers
• Fine line & wrinkle reduction
• Restores youthful appearance
PIGMENTATION SOLUTIONS
• Melasma treatment
• Laser toning
• Depigmentation peels
• Even skin tone
ACNE & SCAR TREATMENTS
• Acne control therapies
• Scar revision
• Microneedling
• Smoother, clearer skin
HAIR RESTORATION (COSMETIC)
• PRP for hair
• Growth boosters
• Scalp rejuvenation
• Improves hair density & quality
BODY CONTOURING
• Fat reduction
• Skin tightening
• Cellulite reduction
• Non-invasive body shaping
3. SURGICAL TREATMENTS (CORRECT, RESTORE & TRANSFORM)
HAIR TRANSPLANT
• FUE / FUT techniques
• Natural-looking results
• Permanent hair restoration
SCAR REVISION SURGERY
• Surgical correction of scars
• Improves texture and appearance
• Restores confidence
RHINOPLASTY (NOSE JOB)
• Reshape nose
• Improves facial harmony
• Functional & aesthetic benefits
BLEPHAROPLASTY (EYE LID SURGERY)
• Removes excess skin and fat
• Reduces puffiness and bags
• Youthful, refreshed look
FACELIFT & CONTOURING SURGERY
• Tightens sagging skin
• Improves facial contours
• Long-lasting anti-aging results
LIPOSUCTION & BODY SCULPTING
• Removes stubborn fat
• Sculpts body shape
• Boosts confidence and appearance
HOW WE CHOOSE THE RIGHT TREATMENT
Detailed consultation & examination
Personalized treatment plan
Safe, effective & evidence-based approach
Best results with minimal downtime
Long-term care & follow-up
OUR PROMISE
Your safety.
Your satisfaction.
Our commitment.
BEAUTY IS PERSONAL. CARE IS PROFESSIONAL.
EXPERT CARE
SAFE TREATMENTS
CUSTOMIZED SOLUTIONS
CONFIDENCE RESTORED
RIGHT TREATMENT. RIGHT TIME. RIGHT RESULTS.
HEALTHY SKIN. STRONG HAIR. HAPPY YOU.

Oral Medications: When Topicals Are Not Enough

Some conditions require treatment from within.

Oral medications may be used for:

Moderate to severe acne
Inflammatory skin diseases
Certain infections
Specific types of hair loss

These treatments can be very effective but require proper supervision.

Monitoring may be needed in some cases.

Hormonal Treatments

Hormonal influence is important in certain conditions.

These treatments may be useful in selected cases such as:

Adult acne
Hair thinning in women
Conditions related to hormonal imbalance

They are not for everyone and require careful evaluation.

Procedural Treatments

Procedures are often used when additional improvement is needed.

Common options include:

Chemical peels
Laser treatments
Microneedling
Light-based therapies

These may help improve pigmentation, acne scars, texture, and sometimes hair density.

Results are gradual and vary between individuals.

Procedures should be performed by trained professionals.

Hair Transplant: A Surgical Option

Hair transplant is considered for certain types of hair loss.

Hair follicles are moved from one part of the scalp to another.

It does not create new hair. It redistributes existing hair.

Results depend on proper selection, technique, and realistic expectations.

It is usually considered after medical treatment.

Newer and Emerging Treatments

New treatments are constantly being introduced.

Some use components from the patient's own blood.

Some use advanced devices.

Some are still under study.

Not all are supported by strong evidence.

It is important to evaluate them carefully.

Safety and Side Effects

Every treatment has benefits and risks.

Even simple creams can cause irritation.

Oral medications may have side effects.

Procedures carry risks if not performed correctly.

Understanding safety is essential.

Realistic Expectations

No treatment works instantly.

Most improvements take time.

Some conditions can be controlled but not completely cured.

Procedures improve appearance but may not give perfect results.

Clear expectations prevent disappointment.

Common Mistakes to Avoid

Using strong treatments without guidance
Stopping treatment too early
Switching treatments frequently
Ignoring side effects
Choosing procedures without proper evaluation

Myth vs Fact

Myth: Stronger treatment works faster.
Fact: Correct treatment works better.

Myth: Procedures give permanent results.
Fact: Many require maintenance.

Myth: If one treatment fails, nothing will work.
Fact: Treatment must be individualized.

Myth: All treatments are safe for everyone.
Fact: Each has specific indications.

Red Flag Warnings

Seek medical advice if you notice:

- Severe side effects
- Worsening symptoms
- Allergic reactions
- No improvement with proper use
- Confusion about treatment

Example: Inconsistent Treatment

A 38-year-old man starts treatment for hair loss but uses it irregularly.

He stops when he does not see immediate results.

Later, when he follows a consistent plan, improvement becomes noticeable.

Consistency is often more important than the treatment itself.

Key Points

Treatment must match the condition.

Topical treatments are usually first.

Oral medications are used when needed.

Procedures provide additional benefit.

Safety and expectations matter.

Chapter Summary

Treatment of skin and hair conditions ranges from simple topical care to advanced procedures. The correct choice depends on the diagnosis, severity, and individual factors.

Understanding treatment options and using them correctly improves outcomes.

Consistency, patience, and proper guidance are essential.

Action Plan

- Understand your diagnosis before starting treatment.
- Begin with simple, appropriate options.
- Use treatments consistently.
- Avoid frequent changes.
- Monitor for side effects.
- Choose procedures carefully.
- Maintain realistic expectations.

Bridge to the Next Chapter

With so many treatments available, it becomes important to separate true scientific progress from marketing claims. In the next chapter, we will explore new research, emerging therapies, and how to avoid confusion.

CHAPTER 21: New Research, Future Treatments, and Industry Hype — Learning to Separate Science from Marketing

A Fast-Changing Field

Skin and hair care is evolving rapidly.

Every year, new treatments, new devices, and new products are introduced. Advertisements promise faster results, better outcomes, and even reversal of aging.

Some of these advances are real and meaningful. Others are exaggerated. A few are simply clever marketing.

For a reader, this creates confusion.

What should you trust?
What is truly effective?
What is still uncertain?

This chapter will help you think clearly and make confident decisions.

What Real Progress Looks Like

True medical progress is usually steady and evidence-based.

In recent years, targeted therapies have improved treatment of certain chronic skin conditions such as psoriasis and severe eczema.

These treatments act on specific pathways in the immune system.

For selected patients, they can provide significant benefit.

This is an example of science leading to real improvement.

Doctor's Pearl

Real advances are supported by consistent evidence, not dramatic promises.

Regenerative Medicine and "Advanced" Therapies

You may hear about treatments that promise regeneration or reversal of damage.

Terms like stem cells and growth factors are often used.

Research in these areas is ongoing and promising in some settings.

However, many treatments marketed under these names are not fully proven.

Not every “advanced” therapy has strong scientific support.

Careful evaluation is important before considering such options.

Artificial Intelligence and Diagnosis

Technology is becoming part of medical care.

Artificial intelligence tools can analyze skin images and assist in diagnosis.

These tools may improve access and early detection in the future.

However, they do not replace clinical judgment.

A doctor considers history, examination, and overall context.

Technology is a tool, not a substitute.

Personalized Skin Care: Promise and Reality

Personalized skin care is a popular concept.

It suggests that products can be tailored to your individual needs.

In theory, this is valuable.

In practice, many products marketed as personalized are based on limited information.

True personalization requires careful evaluation, not just a questionnaire.

Supplements and Popular Trends

Supplements are widely promoted for skin and hair.

Collagen products are popular.

Their benefits are modest and vary between individuals.

Biotin is often recommended for hair growth.

It helps mainly when there is a deficiency.

Most people do not benefit significantly from supplements without a clear need.

Understanding Marketing Language

The skin care industry uses persuasive language.

Terms such as:

Natural
Organic
Chemical-free

Anti-aging
Miracle

These terms sound appealing but are often not scientifically meaningful.

They are designed to attract attention.

Understanding this helps you make better decisions.

How to Evaluate a Claim

A few simple questions can guide you.

Is there consistent evidence behind this claim
Are results realistic or exaggerated
Is safety clearly explained
Is the treatment suitable for your condition

If the answer is unclear, be cautious.

Common Mistakes to Avoid

Trying every new trend
Using multiple new treatments at once
Expecting instant results
Ignoring safety concerns
Spending heavily without clear benefit

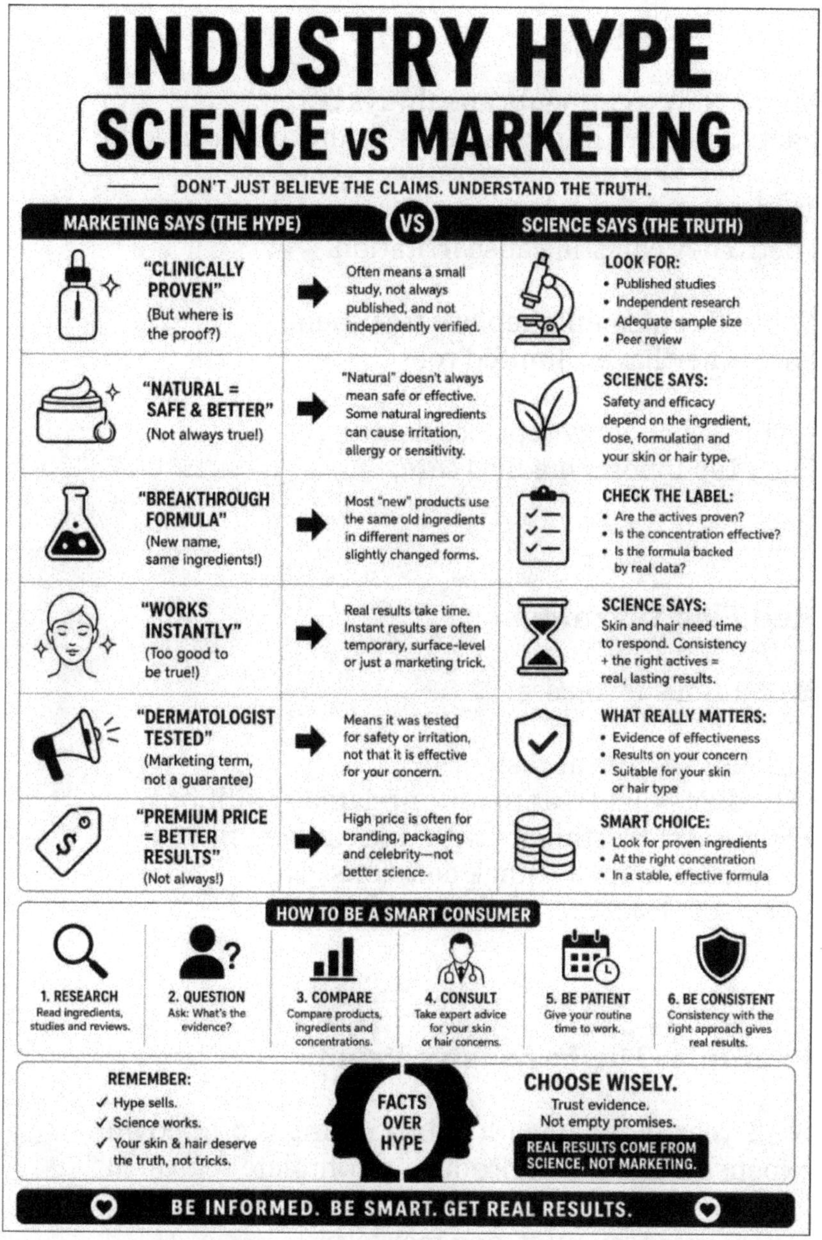
INDUSTRY HYPE
SCIENCE vs MARKETING
DON'T JUST BELIEVE THE CLAIMS. UNDERSTAND THE TRUTH.
MARKETING SAYS (THE HYPE)
VS
SCIENCE SAYS (THE TRUTH)
"CLINICALLY PROVEN" (But where is the proof?)
Often means a small study, not always published, and not independently verified.
LOOK FOR:
• Published studies
• Independent research
• Adequate sample size
• Peer review
"NATURAL = SAFE & BETTER" (Not always true!)
"Natural" doesn't always mean safe or effective. Some natural ingredients can cause irritation, allergy or sensitivity.
SCIENCE SAYS:
Safety and efficacy depend on the ingredient, dose, formulation and your skin or hair type.
"BREAKTHROUGH FORMULA" (New name, same ingredients!)
Most "new" products use the same old ingredients in different names or slightly changed forms.
CHECK THE LABEL:
• Are the actives proven?
• Is the concentration effective?
• Is the formula backed by real data?
"WORKS INSTANTLY" (Too good to be true!)
Real results take time. Instant results are often temporary, surface-level or just a marketing trick.
SCIENCE SAYS:
Skin and hair need time to respond. Consistency + the right actives = real, lasting results.
"DERMATOLOGIST TESTED" (Marketing term, not a guarantee)
Means it was tested for safety or irritation, not that it is effective for your concern.
WHAT REALLY MATTERS:
• Evidence of effectiveness
• Results on your concern
• Suitable for your skin or hair type
"PREMIUM PRICE = BETTER RESULTS" (Not always!)
High price is often for branding, packaging and celebrity—not better science.
SMART CHOICE:
• Look for proven ingredients
• At the right concentration
• In a stable, effective formula
HOW TO BE A SMART CONSUMER
1. RESEARCH
Read ingredients, studies and reviews.
2. QUESTION
Ask: What's the evidence?
3. COMPARE
Compare products, ingredients and concentrations.
4. CONSULT
Take expert advice for your skin or hair concerns.
5. BE PATIENT
Give your routine time to work.
6. BE CONSISTENT
Consistency with the right approach gives real results.
REMEMBER:
✓ Hype sells.
✓ Science works.
✓ Your skin & hair deserve the truth, not tricks.
FACTS OVER HYPE
CHOOSE WISELY.
Trust evidence.
Not empty promises.
REAL RESULTS COME FROM SCIENCE, NOT MARKETING.
BE INFORMED. BE SMART. GET REAL RESULTS.

Myth vs Fact

Myth: New treatments are always better.
Fact: Some are improvements, many are variations.

Myth: Natural products are always safe.
Fact: They can still cause irritation.

Myth: Supplements replace treatment.
Fact: They have a limited role.

Myth: Technology replaces doctors.
Fact: It supports medical care.

Red Flag Warnings

Be cautious if you see:

- Claims of instant results
- Products that treat many unrelated conditions
- High-cost treatments with unclear benefit
- Pressure to make quick decisions
- Lack of clear safety information

Example: The Expensive Promise

A 48-year-old man with hair thinning is offered an expensive treatment promising complete regrowth.

He is convinced by strong marketing.

After treatment, improvement is minimal.

Later, he learns that his condition could have been managed with simpler, evidence-based treatment.

This highlights the importance of careful evaluation.

Key Points

Not all new treatments are proven.

Some represent real progress.

Many claims are exaggerated.

Critical thinking protects you.

Simple, evidence-based care remains the foundation.

Chapter Summary

Advances in skin and hair care continue to emerge. Some provide real benefit, while others are driven by marketing.

Understanding how to evaluate these options helps you make informed decisions.

A balanced approach based on evidence and safety leads to better outcomes.

Action Plan

• Be cautious with new treatments.

• Ask for clear explanation before trying advanced options.

• Focus on proven methods.

• Avoid trying many treatments at once.

• Do not rely solely on supplements.

• Make decisions calmly.

• Seek professional advice when needed.

Bridge to the Next Chapter

Even with good understanding, many practical questions remain in daily life. In the next chapter, we will address the most common questions about skin and hair care in a clear and practical way.

CHAPTER 22: Frequently Asked Questions — Clear Answers to Everyday Doubts

When Simple Questions Create Confusion

Even after understanding causes, treatments, and routines, many questions remain.

Patients often ask the same practical doubts in different ways.

Should I wash my face twice or three times?
Is sunscreen really needed every day?
Why is my hair falling even after using good products?
Do supplements help?
Am I doing something wrong?

These are not trivial questions. They reflect confusion created by mixed advice.

In this chapter, I will answer these questions the way I do in the clinic, simply and honestly.

Daily Skin Care Questions

How often should I wash my face?
For most people, once or twice daily is enough. More frequent washing can damage the skin barrier and lead to dryness or irritation.

Do I need separate morning and night routines?
Yes, but keep it simple. Morning care focuses on protection, especially sunscreen. Night care focuses on cleansing and repair.

Can I skip moisturizer if my skin is oily?
No. Oily skin also needs hydration. Skipping moisturizer may increase oil production.

Is sunscreen really necessary every day?
Yes. Daily exposure to sunlight contributes to aging, pigmentation, and long-term skin damage.

Hair Care Questions

How often should I wash my hair?
There is no single rule. Oily scalp may need frequent washing. Dry or sensitive scalp may need less frequent washing.

Does washing cause hair loss?
No. It removes hair that is already shedding.

Do hair oils help hair growth?
They improve dryness and shine. They do not treat most causes of hair loss.

Should I brush my hair frequently?
Gentle brushing is fine. Excessive brushing can damage hair.

Hair Loss Concerns

When should I worry about hair loss?
If you notice sudden heavy shedding, patchy hair loss, or gradual thinning that continues over time.

Will my hair grow back?
In many cases, yes, especially when the cause is temporary. Some conditions require treatment.

Do supplements help hair growth?
Only when there is a deficiency.

Acne and Skin Problems

Why is my acne not improving?
Acne treatment takes time. It may take several weeks or months to show improvement. Consistency is essential.

Does diet affect acne?
It may influence acne in some individuals, but the effect varies.

Should I squeeze pimples?
No. It increases the risk of infection and scarring.

Pigmentation and Aging

Can dark spots be removed completely?
Some improve significantly, but complete removal may not always be possible.

Do anti-aging creams work?
Some help improve appearance gradually. Results are modest.

Can aging be prevented?
No. It can be slowed but not stopped.

Products and Treatments

How do I choose the right product?
Choose based on your skin type and problem, not on marketing claims.

Can I use many active products together?
It is better to introduce one at a time to avoid irritation.

How long should I try a product?
Usually several weeks before judging its effectiveness.

When Should I See a Doctor

When should I seek medical advice?
If symptoms are persistent, worsening, or unclear.

Are all skin problems serious?
Most are not, but some need evaluation.

Can I treat everything at home?
No. Some conditions require proper diagnosis and treatment.

Doctor's Pearl

Simple understanding prevents unnecessary confusion and expense.

Common Mistakes to Avoid

Relying only on internet advice
Changing products too frequently
Expecting quick results
Ignoring warning signs
Overusing treatments

Myth vs Fact

Myth: Good skin requires many products.
Fact: Simple routines often work better.

Myth: Hair loss is always permanent.
Fact: Many types are manageable.

Myth: Expensive products are more effective.
Fact: Correct choice matters more.

Red Flag Warnings

Seek medical advice if you notice:

- Persistent or worsening symptoms
- Sudden hair loss
- Changing skin lesions
- Severe itching or rash
- Signs of infection

Example: Too Much Advice, Too Little Clarity

A 48-year-old woman follows multiple online routines and uses several products.

Her skin becomes irritated.

When she simplifies her routine and uses targeted treatment, her skin improves.

This highlights the importance of clarity over complexity.

Key Points

Most common questions have simple answers.

Consistency matters more than complexity.

Understanding reduces confusion.

Professional advice helps when needed.

Chapter Summary

Many skin and hair concerns arise from confusion and mixed information. This chapter addresses common questions in a practical and straightforward manner.

A simple, consistent approach works best. When problems persist or worsen, medical evaluation is important.

Clarity leads to better decisions.

Action Plan

• Keep your routine simple.

• Avoid frequent changes.

• Be patient with results.

• Seek clarity before trying new treatments.

• Watch for warning signs.

• Consult a doctor when needed.

Bridge to the Final Chapter

You now have the knowledge. In the final chapter, we will bring everything together into a simple, practical plan that you can follow for life.

CHAPTER 23: Your Lifelong Skin and Hair Health Plan — Simple Habits, Lasting Results

From Information to Action

You have now reached the most important part of this book.

You have learned about skin structure, hair growth, common problems, warning signs, diagnosis, treatments, and modern trends.

But knowledge alone does not change outcomes.

What changes outcomes is what you do every day.

This chapter brings everything together into a clear, practical plan you can follow for life.

Not complicated. Not expensive. Not time-consuming.

Just thoughtful, consistent care.

The Core Principle: Consistency Over Complexity

Most people start with enthusiasm.

They buy several products. They follow detailed routines. They expect visible improvement quickly.

Then life becomes busy. The routine becomes irregular. Products are changed. Results become inconsistent.

The truth is simple.

You do not need a perfect routine.

You need a consistent one.

Small steps done regularly are more powerful than complex routines done occasionally.

Doctor's Pearl

The best routine is the one you can follow every day.

Your Daily Routine: Clear and Practical

Morning

Cleanse gently if needed
Apply a suitable moisturizer
Use sunscreen on exposed areas

Night

Cleanse to remove dirt and oil
Apply moisturizer
Use a targeted treatment if required

This simple structure works for most people.

Weekly Care: Thoughtful, Not Excessive

Gentle exfoliation if suitable
Hair conditioning as needed
Check your skin for any new or changing lesions
Observe your hair pattern and scalp condition

There is no need for daily complex treatments.

Lifestyle Habits That Matter

Skin and hair health reflect daily living.

Balanced nutrition with adequate protein
Regular sleep for repair
Stress management
Regular physical activity
Sun protection

These habits support long-term health.

Product Use: Keep It Focused

Choose products based on your specific need.

Avoid using multiple strong ingredients together.

Introduce new products slowly.

Stop products that irritate your skin.

Simple routines often give better results.

When to Seek Medical Care

Some problems require professional attention.

Persistent acne
Unexplained hair loss
Changing moles
Severe itching
Recurrent infections

Early evaluation prevents complications.

Realistic Expectations: The Key to Satisfaction

No treatment works overnight.

Most improvements take weeks or months.

Some conditions can be controlled but not completely cured.

Procedures improve appearance but may not create perfection.

Understanding this prevents disappointment.

Common Mistakes to Avoid

Changing routines frequently
Using too many products
Ignoring warning signs
Expecting quick results
Stopping treatment too early

Avoiding these mistakes improves outcomes.

Myth vs Fact

Myth: Expensive products give better results.
Fact: Correct products matter more than cost.

Myth: Hair loss cannot be managed.
Fact: Many types can be controlled.

Myth: More treatment gives faster results.
Fact: Over-treatment causes harm.

Red Flag Warnings

Seek medical advice if you notice:

- Changing moles or lesions
- Persistent symptoms
- Sudden hair loss
- Severe itching or infection
- Symptoms affecting daily life

Example: The Power of Simplicity

A 54-year-old woman had dry skin and gradual hair thinning.

She used multiple products without benefit.

When she simplified her routine, improved her diet, managed stress, and followed a consistent plan, her condition improved steadily.

This is not unusual.

Simple, steady care works.

Key Points

Consistency matters more than perfection.

Simple routines are effective.

Lifestyle habits play a major role.

Early attention prevents complications.

Patience is essential.

Chapter Summary

Long-term skin and hair health depends on simple, consistent habits. A basic daily routine, appropriate product use, healthy lifestyle, and early attention to warning signs form the foundation.

Complex routines and frequent changes often do more harm than good.

A calm, steady approach leads to better results.

Action Plan

- Follow a simple daily routine.
- Use products suited to your needs.
- Protect your skin from sun exposure.
- Maintain balanced nutrition.
- Sleep well and manage stress.
- Observe changes early.
- Seek medical advice when needed.
- Stay consistent and patient.

Final Thoughts

Skin and hair care should not be confusing.

With the right understanding, it becomes simple, practical, and manageable.

Your goal is not perfection.

Your goal is healthy, comfortable skin and confident living.

Bridge to Appendices

In the appendices that follow, you will find simple checklists, practical tools, and a 30-day plan to help you apply everything you have learned in your daily life.

APPENDIX 1: Daily Skin and Hair Care Checklist — Keep It Simple, Keep It Consistent

A Routine You Can Actually Follow

Most people do not fail because they lack information.

They fail because their routine is too complicated to maintain.

This checklist is designed to be practical. You should be able to follow it even on your busiest days.

Morning Routine

- Wash your face gently if needed
- Pat dry, do not rub
- Apply a suitable moisturizer
- Apply sunscreen on face, neck, and exposed areas
- Comb hair gently
- Avoid tight hairstyles
- Drink adequate fluids

Evening Routine

- Cleanse your skin to remove dirt and oil
- Apply moisturizer
- Use prescribed or targeted treatment if needed

- Comb hair gently
- Avoid sleeping with tight hairstyles

Weekly Care

- Gentle exfoliation if suitable
- Condition hair as needed
- Clean combs and brushes
- Check your skin for new or changing lesions
- Observe hair and scalp

Simple Reminders

- Keep your routine simple
- Be consistent
- Avoid frequent product changes
- Give time for results

APPENDIX 2: Ingredient Guide — What Helps, What Needs Caution

A Practical Way to Understand Products

You do not need to remember long ingredient lists.

Focus on what works, what needs caution, and what is often overhyped.

Common Helpful Ingredients

Retinoids — help acne and aging
Niacinamide — supports barrier and reduces redness
Hyaluronic acid — improves hydration
Ceramides — repair the skin barrier
Salicylic acid — helps acne
Benzoyl peroxide — reduces acne bacteria
Sunscreen agents — protect from sun damage

Hair-Related Ingredients

Minoxidil — helps certain types of hair loss
Ketoconazole — helps dandruff and scalp inflammation
Conditioning agents — improve hair texture

Use with Caution

Strong exfoliating acids
Fragrances
Alcohol-heavy products
Frequent chemical treatments

Often Overhyped

"Miracle" anti-aging claims
Instant results
"Chemical-free" labels
Products claiming to treat many unrelated problems

Doctor's Pearl

Choose products based on your problem, not on marketing.

APPENDIX 3: Red Flag Symptoms – When You Should Not Wait

Early Action Prevents Bigger Problems

Do not ignore these signs.

- A mole that changes in size, shape, or color
- A sore that does not heal
- Sudden or patchy hair loss
- Severe or persistent itching
- Rapidly spreading rash
- Signs of infection such as redness, swelling, or pus
- Yellowing of skin or eyes
- Recurrent infections
- Thickening or unusual discoloration of skin

Important Reminder

If something persists or worsens, it deserves attention.

APPENDIX 4: 30-Day Skin and Hair Health Plan — A Practical Start

A Step-by-Step Approach

This plan helps you move from confusion to clarity.

Week 1: Reset

- Stop unnecessary products
- Start gentle cleansing and moisturizing
- Begin daily sunscreen
- Observe your skin and hair

Week 2: Build Routine

- Continue daily routine
- Improve diet and hydration
- Avoid known triggers
- Begin simple stress management

Week 3: Add Targeted Care

- Introduce one treatment if needed
- Monitor response
- Continue lifestyle habits

Week 4: Maintain and Adjust

- Continue routine
- Review progress
- Adjust if needed
- Plan long-term care

Final Tips

- Be patient
- Stay consistent
- Avoid over-treatment
- Seek help when needed

APPENDIX 5: Preparing for a Doctor Visit — Make It Effective

Use Your Time Wisely

A good consultation saves time, money, and frustration.

Before the Visit

- Write down your main concern
- Note when it started
- List all products and medications
- Identify possible triggers
- Note any other symptoms

During the Visit

- Be clear and honest
- Ask questions
- Understand the diagnosis
- Clarify the treatment plan

After the Visit

- Follow treatment consistently
- Do not stop early
- Observe response
- Schedule follow-up if needed

Closing Note

Healthy skin and hair are not built by quick fixes.

They are built by understanding, simple habits, and steady care.

With the right approach, you move from confusion to clarity, and from frustration to confidence.

Thank You and Please Review the Book

Thank you for taking the time to read this book. I sincerely hope it has helped you understand your health a little more clearly and has given you practical, everyday steps you can follow with confidence. If you found this book helpful, **I would truly appreciate it if you could leave a brief and honest review.** Even a few lines sharing your experience can make a meaningful difference. Your feedback helps other readers find reliable, trustworthy health information and supports them in making better decisions for themselves and their families.

Warm regards,

Dr Prabhat Das

Continue your Healthcare Journey with these Books

Good health is a journey, not a single step. It is not achieved in one day or with one book. That is why I created the "Better Health with Dr Das Series", with each book addressing a different common condition. If you would like easy, practical guidance on other everyday health concerns, you may wish to explore the rest of books in this series.

Books in this series:

- Better Health starts Here: A Doctor's Guide to Staying Healthy After 40
- A Doctor's Easy Guide to Understanding & Managing OBESITY
- Doctor, What DIET Is Best for Me?
- Doctor, Why Can't I Lose Weight? A Doctor's Guide to Safe & Sustainable Weight Loss)
- A Doctor's Easy Guide to GLP-1 for Obesity
- A Doctor's Easy Guide to Understanding & Managing HIGH BLOOD PRESSURE
- A Doctor's Guide to Living Well With DIABETES
- A Doctor's Guide to Understanding & Managing THYROID DISEASES
- A Doctor's Guide to Understanding & Managing HIGH CHOLESTEROL
- A Doctor's Practical Guide to HEART HEALTH After 40: How to Protect Your Heart & Live Longer
- A Doctor's Guide to Healing & Reversing FATTY LIVER DISEASE: Simple, Natural & Science-Based Steps to Reduce Liver Fat and Prevent Complications

- Control Your ACID REFLUX, HEARTBURN & GERD: A Doctor's Practical Guide that Works
- Live Comfortably with IRRITABLE BOWEL SYNDROME: A Doctor's Practical Guide to Understanding & Managing IBS
- A Doctor's Practical Guide to Understanding & Managing GALLBLADDER STONES & OTHER PROBLEMS
- Take Control of COPD: A Doctor's Practical Guide to Better Breathing
- Living Better with ASTHMA: A Doctor's Practical Guide to Asthma Control
- SLEEP APNEA, INSOMNIA & OTHER SLEEP DISORDERS: A Doctor's Practical Guide to Better Sleep & Better Health
- Protect Your KIDNEYS: A Doctor's Practical Guide to Kidney Health & Prevention
- PROSTATE HEALTH: A Doctor's Practical Guide to Early Detection & Care
- ARTHRITIS: A Doctor's Practical Guide to Pain Control & Mobility
- STROKE: A Doctor's Practical Guide to Prevention & Early detection
- HEART ATTACK: A Doctor's Practical Guide to Prevention & Early detection
- CANCER: A Doctor's Practical Guide to Prevention & Early detection
- BACK PAIN: A Doctor's Practical Guide that Works
- SKIN & HAIR CARE: A Doctor's Practical Guide to Healthy Skin & Hair
- DEMENTIA & MEMORY LOSS: A Doctor's Practical Guide to Prevention & Management
- Doctor, Why Am I TIRED All the Time? Fixing Fatigue & Getting Your Energy Back

www.ingramcontent.com/pod-product-compliance
Lightning Source LLC
Chambersburg PA
CBHW060135011026
52423CB00003B/29
* 9 7 8 1 9 7 1 6 7 2 7 6 2 *